PSYCHIATRIC
PEARLS

PSYCHIATRIC PEARLS

JEFFREY M. LYNESS, MD

Assistant Professor of Psychiatry
Director, Psychiatry Clerkship
University of Rochester School of
Medicine and Dentistry
Rochester, New York

Clinical Director
Geriatrics and Neuropsychiatry Unit
Strong Memorial Hospital
Rochester, New York

F. A. DAVIS COMPANY • Philadelphia

F. A. Davis Company
1915 Arch Street
Philadelphia, PA 19103

Printed in the United States of America

Last digit indicates print number: 10 9 8 7 6 5 4 3 2 1

Senior Medical Editor: Robert W. Reinhardt
Developmental Editor: Bernice M. Wissler
Production Editor: Jessica Howie Martin
Cover Designer: Louis J. Forgione

Library of Congress Cataloging-in-Publication Data

Lyness, Jeffrey M., 1960–
    Psychiatric pearls / Jeffrey M. Lyness.
        p.   cm.
    Includes index.
    ISBN 0-8036-0280-4 (paper)
    1. Psychiatry—Handbooks, manuals, etc.   I. Title.
    [DNLM: 1. Mental Disorders—diagnosis.   2. Mental
Disorders—therapy.   3. Psychiatry—methods.
WM 141 L988p 1997]
RC456.L96   1997
616.89—DC21
DNLM/DLC
for Library of Congress   96-29495
                                                         CIP

As new scientific information becomes available through basic and clinical research, recommended treatments and drug therapies undergo changes. The author and publisher have done everything possible to make this book accurate, up to date, and in accord with accepted standards at the time of publication. The author, editors, and publisher are not responsible for errors or omissions or for consequences from application of the book, and make no warranty, expressed or implied, in regard to the contents of the book. Any practice described in this book should be applied by the reader in accordance with professional standards of care used in regard to the unique circumstances that may apply in each situation. The reader is advised always to check product information (package inserts) for changes and new information regarding dose and contraindications before administering any drug. Caution is especially urged when using new or infrequently ordered drugs.

Preface

Welcome to your psychiatry experience! Whatever your previous exposure to the field (in many cases, probably none!), you have no doubt heard many things about psychiatry and psychiatric patients. Some of these things may have been pejorative. Others may lead you to worry that you are about to encounter situations that are strange, anxiety-provoking, frightening, or even dangerous. In fact, there *are* some important differences between your work in psychiatric settings and that in other clinical medicine settings. Learning about these differences is part of the objectives of the rotation. You will be relieved to discover that most work in this field is highly parallel to work in other medical settings. You'll also discover that, after a week or so of settling in (as on other rotations), you will feel clearer about your roles and tasks. If you're like most trainees, you'll soon feel comfortable with—nay, even look forward to—coming to work. Such comfort and enjoyment will stem from the inherent interestingness of the patients and their disorders (not to mention from the brilliance, enthusiasm, and niceness of your teachers) and will greatly facilitate your learning and your ability to interact positively with your patients and colleagues.

The goal of this book, then, is to help you to reach more rapidly the point of feeling competent and comfortable. The choice of topics, or more precisely the approach to these topics, is modeled on what students have found important in the running of our third-year medical student psychiatry clerkship. This book will also be relevant to other physician trainees newly joining a psychiatry service, whether they be brand new psychiatry residents or residents from another specialty taking an elective. This book may also be useful to the many non-physician professional trainees who work in psychiatric settings, parallelling the critical roles played by many disciplines in delivering care to the mentally ill.

In this book we consider aspects of the psychiatry rotation itself, including goals, logistics, and approaches to productive and successful clerkship performance. We examine the basics en route to mastering the knowledge base and skills you'll be working on during the rotation. We also discuss the framework within which psychiatric care is rendered, including comments on settings and the people who inhabit them.

Please note that this book is intended as an introductory guide. It is neither a textbook nor a reference work, both of which you will need access to during the rotation. Rather, it is best digested whole at the very beginning of the experience, perhaps the evening before you start the rotation. You may find it useful to refer back to it occasionally early in the rotation, but if this book achieves its goal, you will rapidly progress beyond it as you settle into your work. (Talk about planned obsolescence . . .)

I would like to thank Drs. Melissa DelBello and Eric D. Caine for "making" me write this book; Drs. Yeates Conwell, Laurence Guttmacher, and Mary Lou Meyers for reviewing the manuscript; and the many students and residents who have stimulated and nurtured my development as a teacher.

Jeffrey M. Lyness, MD
Rochester, New York

Contents

1
PART

How to Think Psychiatrically

These first three chapters are intended to orient you to the field of psychiatry. I'll begin by defining some basic terms—*psychiatry*, for example. (When I said "basic" terms, I meant it!) Next, we'll consider the process of diagnostic reasoning in psychiatry and how it's both similar to and different from what you've been doing in other medical specialties. Finally, we'll reacquaint ourselves with some of the theoretical frameworks useful to psychiatric formulation, remembering that the basic sciences of all clinical work encompass not only biomedical but also psychological and psychosocial perspectives.

1

CHAPTER

Introduction

WHAT IS PSYCHIATRY?

Psychiatry is the branch of medicine concerned with the diagnosis and treatment of persons with mental disorders. Like other medical specialties, it is both an applied science and a craft (or an art, depending on one's perspective). Psychiatry draws on a variety of basic sciences including numerous aspects of neurobiology, psychological theories (which themselves include a variety of perspectives), and on psychosocial theories (which include several interpersonal, family, cultural, legal, and ethical perspectives). *Psychiatrists* are physicians who have completed specialty residency training in psychiatry. Many other professionals contribute to the care of patients with psychiatric disorders; some further descriptions of them and their roles are found in Chapter 17.

Of course, the above definition assumes that we're clear on what we mean by the term *mental disorders*. And, unfortunately, there is room for ambiguity and debate about both the "mental" and "disorder" parts of the term. At the risk of oversimplification, for these purposes we'll think of "mental" as referring to thoughts, feelings, and actions, regardless of what we know or don't know about the relationship of these things to brain function. "Disorder," in this context, refers to a difficulty that is manifested by subjective distress, observable dysfunction or disability, or both. Let's assume, then, that mental disorders are troubles involving thoughts, feelings, or actions. What these troubles are and how to diagnose and treat them are, of course, a large part of what you're here to learn.

WHY SHOULD I LEARN ANY PSYCHIATRY?

Assuming that you're undecided as to choice of specialty, or that you have already decided on a specialty other than psychiatry, you've probably asked yourself some version of this question. (I hope with a tone of curiosity rather than resentment). Let's start with the overall objectives of the rotation. These boil down to three major realms: developing interpersonal technical competence, learning the basics of the diagnosis and treatment of psychopathology, and learning biopsychosocial integration.

Interpersonal Technical Competence

All physicians need to develop their skills in interacting with patients and families because the doctor-patient relationship is the *primary* tool for gathering data and initiating therapeutic interventions in all clinical specialties (as you were surely taught earlier in medical school). Psychiatry is a particularly good field in which to develop these skills. For one thing, you'll be working directly with professionals who are highly knowledgeable and skilled regarding doctor-patient relationship issues. Discussion of these issues is central to most psychiatric settings. Therefore, you will be able to get feedback about patient interviews, family meetings, and difficult interactions with patients to a degree that may not be true of most of your other rotations. And the patient populations will also give you a highly concentrated experience, under close supervision, with the difficult interactions that you will certainly face time and time again in all branches of clinical medicine—for example, patients who are mute, withdrawn, or angry; patients who are unable to communicate well because of cognitive or psychotic symptoms; circumstances in which you and the patient (and/or the family) disagree about diagnosis or treatment plan; poor compliance with treatment recommendations; dealing with the effects of chronic illness and disability; delivering bad news about a diagnosis or prognosis; and recognizing both the powers and the limitations we as physicians have working with our patients. The skills and ways of critically thinking about these issues that you learn on your psychiatry rotation will enrich and complement your clinical experiences throughout your career.

Learning About Psychopathology

All physicians need to understand the basics of the diagnosis and treatment of psychopathology. Why?

- Mental disorders are extremely *common*. Some, such as depression or alcohol dependence, have greater point and lifetime prevalence than almost any physical disorder you could name.

- These disorders *matter*. They cause or contribute to functional disability—as measured in real terms—for example, time lost from work and days spent in bed. The enormous degree to which they contribute to functional disability is comparable to that associated with major chronic physical illnesses such as cardiovascular diseases.
- Psychiatric treatments *work*. Recent large-scale reviews conducted under the auspices of the National Institutes of Health conclude that treatments for the major psychiatric disorders are at least as effective, and as well supported by scientific evidence, as treatments for most major physical diseases.
- Most patients with psychiatric disorders never seek care from the "official" mental health system, but they do see other medical providers, including primary care physicians and specialists. Thus, no matter what your clinical field, you will see plenty of patients with psychiatric symptoms. (Indeed, most estimates suggest that psychiatric symptoms and disorders are the sole factor or a substantial contributing factor underlying most doctor visits.) Moreover, it is mostly up to nonpsychiatric physicians to ensure that these people get the help that they (and society) need.

Learning Biopsychosocial Integration

All clinicians routinely encounter and use a wide variety of data in planning treatment. These data may include details of physical symptoms, physical examination and laboratory findings, behavioral observations of patients and families (including mental status examination), and information about social services and other community resources. Pulling these data together is essential to patient care, and, in fact, physicians all *do* this. Yet in many of the acute medical settings that still form the bulk of most trainees' experiences, biomedical data receive the most emphasis in both formal and informal teaching sessions. Psychological and psychosocial data are too often left unstated, as if they are either unimportant or an unteachable part of the nebulous art of medicine. In fact, these types of data are critical to patient care, and it is quite possible to learn how to gather such information systematically and combine it with other clinical data as part of formulating patient problems and creating a comprehensive treatment plan. Modeling and teaching how to do this can and should occur in all clinical settings, but psychiatry is a particularly good place to do so because explicit attention to the mental status examination, psychological and family system formulations, and other psychosocial issues is part of the specialty's expertise and values.

BEGINNING YOUR ROTATION

The basic ground rules for getting off to a good start on your psychiatry rotation are the same as they are for any clerkship. (Except that for this one, you've already taken a magnificent first step by reading this book.) Make sure you understand the mechanics and logistics of the rotation as quickly as possible. The sooner you're clear on where you need to be when, the faster you can move on to the harder stuff—the goals and objectives. What are the bodies of material you need to learn, and what texts and other references will you use? What skills will you be developing? What supervision is available to help you? And what is your role in the clinical settings of the rotation? The question of roles is often subtle and difficult to resolve simply by referring to your clerkship syllabus or texts. It also may be particularly hard for you at first because of the complex multidisciplinary team approach used in many psychiatry settings (see Chap. 17). Paying attention to cues and feedback, explicit and implicit, and being conscious that role performance is a crucial part of your job as a clinical clerk will help immensely.

You should receive feedback from your teachers throughout the clerkship. Most assuredly, you will receive some final summative evaluation at the end, which in most medical schools consists of both a narrative description of your performance and a final grade. There's enough variability among schools to make it impossible to comment specifically on grading here. But, in a general way, evaluations will comment on the following aspects of your performance:

- Academically, how much do you know? What skills do you demonstrate in reviewing and synthesizing information to expand your knowledge base in relevant areas? How well do you apply new knowledge to clinical reasoning?
- Clinically, how well are you able to gather patient-related data, organize it for written or oral presentation, and formulate a thoughtful differential diagnosis and management plan? At what level are your procedural skills (which for psychiatry will particularly emphasize mental status examination and interview skills with patients and families)?
- Interpersonally, how well do you work with your peers, teachers, and other colleagues? To what extent do you convey the following

characteristics: enthusiasm and energy for the subject matter, patient care, and your own education; professionalism, a vague but important concept that may be inferred by your teachers from attire, grooming, demeanor, and a sense of your level of maturity, responsibility, and integrity; assertiveness, enough that you seek out an active role with your patients and your coworkers, yet balanced with a knowledge of your own limitations, so that you don't take on more than you can handle; and receptivity to feedback.

2
CHAPTER

Differential Diagnosis

Constructing a differential diagnosis is just as important in psychiatry as it is in the rest of medicine, for much the same reasons—the diagnosis will have important implications for prognosis and treatment. Particularly since the publication of the *Diagnostic and Statistical Manual of Mental Disorders*, 3rd edition *(DSM-III)* in 1980, and on through its descendants (the most recent being *DSM-IV*), the use of specific diagnostic criteria has become widespread in psychiatry. This use has made possible the explosion of empiric research that allows us to state that the treatment of psychiatric conditions is soundly based on scientific evidence.

Yet it is important to recognize that there is much that psychiatric (and other medical) diagnoses do not tell us about our patients. Whether our patient has newly diagnosed schizophrenia, systemic lupus erythematosus, or atherosclerotic heart disease, we can state the broad range of possible disease courses, and we know the most common courses, but we cannot predict with certainty how our specific patient will do over time. The same is true regarding treatment: We know what classes of medications or what types of psychosocial interventions may be of help, but we do not know which specific ones will prove most effective in a given patient until we try them. Also, psychiatric diagnoses in and of themselves don't tell us any more about the person who has the disorder than most medical diagnoses. Personality disorders are a partial exception, but even here the diagnosis barely scratches the surface.

Many students, and for that matter, some experienced psychiatrists, criticize DSM-style diagnoses for these limitations, but they are limitations inherent to any diagnostic system. To put it more positively, we must recognize the genuine advantages of psychiatric diagnostic thinking. At the same time, we should recognize that we must know enormous amounts of clinical data in addition to the diagnosis to effectively interact with, make prognoses, and treat our patients.

There is, however, one fundamental difference in the diagnostic process in psychiatry versus in the rest of medicine (Fig. 2–1). Most medical diagnoses are defined by a specific etiology—for example, an abnormal gene or an infectious agent—or by a specific pathoanatomy or pathophysiology—for example, a high prevalence of immature cells on bone marrow biopsy or altered metabolic function caused by insulin deficiency. Therefore, standard clinical reasoning has you gather data—symptoms, signs, laboratory tests—into recognizable syndromes (symptom clusters). Each specific syndrome then leads to an etiologic or pathophysiological diagnosis. For instance, a patient presents to you with dyspnea, a symptom that suggests a rather broad range of diagnoses. On questioning, you learn that the patient also has orthopnea, paroxysmal nocturnal dyspnea, and swollen ankles. You already recognize a symptom cluster that is strongly suggestive of congestive heart failure. Further gathering of data reveals stigmata on physical examination, and chest X ray and arterial blood gas confirm the presence of congestive heart failure. This physio-

- There are no simple one-to-one relationships between psychiatric syndromes and their causes (actual or putative). One syndrome may have numerous etiologies (Fig. 2–2A). For instance, a major depressive syndrome may be due to (idiopathic) major depressive disorder, (idiopathic) bipolar disorder, (idiopathic) schizoaffective disorder, normal bereavement, hypothyroidism, excessive alcohol intake, Parkinson's disease, anemia, or any of dozens of other possible explanations. Conversely, one etiology may manifest as any of several psychiatric syndromes (Fig. 2–2B). As examples, hypothyroidism may present as a depressive syndrome, dementia, delirium, or mania (myxedema madness); a frontal lobe brain tumor may present with psychosis, depression, mania, dementia, or personality changes.

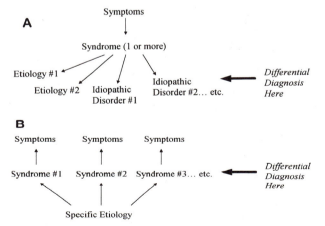

Figure 2–2. Diagnostic reasoning in psychiatry. *(A)* Etiologic differential diagnosis. *(B)* Syndromic differential diagnosis.

So we see that tracing a simple line from symptoms to syndrome to a single etiologically based diagnosis isn't going to work very well. What to do? In effect, you need to construct *two* parallel differential diagnoses, one at the level of the putative etiology (pathophysiology) and the other at the level of the syndrome.

- At the level of pathophysiology (see Fig. 2–2A):
  - Does the patient have any evident systemic physiologic conditions that might contribute to psychiatric syndromes?
  - Which conditions might contribute to which syndromes? For example, anemia of recent onset might contribute to a new-onset major depressive syndrome but would not explain the same patient's life-long obsessions and compulsions.

- At the syndromic level (see Fig. 2–2B):
  - Does the patient have a psychotic syndrome, and if so, can it be characterized further (e.g., nonbizarre delusions only, or bizarre delusions plus auditory hallucinations plus thought blocking)?
  - Does the patient have a mood syndrome? Is it manic, major depressive, mixed, or a "lesser" syndrome such as hypomania or dysthymia?
  - Does the patient have a cognitive deficit syndrome? If so, is it a delirium, dementia, or amnestic syndrome?
  - Does the patient have anxiety symptoms, and if so, does he or she follow the pattern of specific anxiety syndromes such as panic attacks, post-traumatic stress syndromes, or obsessions or compulsions?
  - Does the patient have other psychiatric syndromes (e.g., enduring dysfunction of personality or eating-disordered behaviors, for instance)?

- Do any of the above syndromes coexist (e.g., manic psychosis or delirium with a depressive syndrome)?

Of course, this is only a start toward establishing a definitive diagnosis. *DSM-IV* diagnoses begin with syndromic criteria being met. But then additional factors come into play. What has been the course of this syndrome over time? Has this syndrome ever coexisted in the past with additional syndromes, such as major depressive syndrome with a delusional syndrome or panic attacks? How has the syndrome affected the patient's functional status, and how has this changed over time?

Answering these questions may not be easy, and, in fact, definitive diagnosis may require considerable time—time to gather data from a variety of sources and time to observe the patient's symptoms and course. More thoughts on data-gathering are presented in Chapter 11 on the psychiatric workup. We will now turn to an overview of theoretical notions underlying the psychiatric diagnostic process.

3
CHAPTER

All Those Theories

Theoretical notions in psychiatry seem at best a muddled mess to many trainees new to the field. It appears that most disorders don't have a known cause that is proven by scientific methods and is quantifiable or directly observable like those of most self-respecting medical disorders. And, so the legend goes, in an attempt to cover up their ignorance, mental health professionals invent a confusing array of pseudojargon, often charmingly referred to in the lay press as "psychobabble." So what's a medical student or resident, fresh off his or her internal medicine or general surgery rotation, to do when faced with this unacceptable mass of obfuscation?

Well, for starters, let's take a step back from this "legend" and put things in proper perspective. Sure, as we discussed in the last chapter, most psychiatric disorders are idiopathic. But just because a disorder is idiopathic doesn't mean we can't describe its clinical phenomenology, course, or treatment responsiveness—and again, the empirical clinical studies of, say, bipolar disorder are comparable in quality to those of other idiopathic conditions such as rheumatoid arthritis.

It is true that etiologic theories abound for

most idiopathic disorders. You can view this as confusing or as part of what makes medicine and psychiatry intellectually challenging and fun. It is also true that mental health has attracted more than its share of untested notions, fringe movements, and publicity seekers using their idiosyncratic ideas as an intended springboard to fortune or fame. But the rest of medicine has its own long and equally dishonorable traditions of, shall we say, alternative treatments unsupported by evidence. (This is aside from mainstream treatments unsupported by rigorous evidence, a greater proportion of the practice of medicine than most physicians wish to admit.) Just as in medicine, there are core concepts in psychiatry that are generally agreed upon, supported by evidence, and useful. You can and will master these ideas, and the fringe stuff won't intrude on your work any more than faddish notions of "total environmental allergy" will affect your work in pulmonary medicine or the allergy/immunology clinic.

As a prelude to examining some specific theories, let's consider four broader issues. The first is the notion, alluded to before, that pathophysiology must be construed broadly to include more than just the processes considered by traditional pathology and physiology. For example, we all know that the cause of cholera is *Vibrio cholerae*, and that its pathophysiology involves an enterotoxin's effects on electrolyte flow across intestinal mucosa, producing a secretory diarrhea. Yet, from a psychosocial perspective, the pathogenesis of cholera epidemics involves societal conditions, such as a contaminated water supply, that allow the growth and rapid distribution of the *Vibrio* bacillus to large numbers of persons. Indeed, the most effective treatment for cholera, namely the prevention of epidemics by revamping the water supply, was successfully implemented in industrialized cities such as London in the mid-1800s, long before anyone had heard of bacilli (let alone cyclic AMP). The most common and important psychiatric disorders rarely occur in true epidemics, but attention to psychological and psychosocial "pathogenesis" remains essential.

The second point is that more than one theory may be invoked simultaneously to help understand a patient's disorder. This is so for two reasons: The disorder may truly be multifactorial as in the "28% genetic, 31% developmental" example given in Chapter 2. Also, different theories may shed important perspectives on what is essentially the same thing. For example, a small child frequently separated from parents may develop unconscious fears that are expressed in adult life as panic attacks; thus, we have a developmentally based psychodynamic approach to this person's symptoms. At the same time, however, we might recognize that the frequent separations also led to an increase in the activity or sensitivity of certain neuroanatomic pathways, such as the noradrenergic projections of the locus coeruleus, and that hyperactivity of these systems underlies our patient's panic attacks. These perspectives—and others that might be added—in effect describe different views of the same elephant, and all must be considered to achieve the deepest understanding of the patient's distress and to consider the full range of possible treatment options.

Third, treatment modalities also affect multiple levels of conceptual organization simultaneously. Thus, just because antidepressant medications work for depression doesn't mean that depression is entirely a "brain" disease. The medications ameliorate ideational and affective symptoms, as much as somatic symptoms, of depression. At the same time, psychosocial treatments also work for most patients with major depression.

Finally, theories that help us understand a disorder don't necessarily lead to effective treatments. For example, psychodynamics gives us a rich perspective from which to understand the symptoms of obsessive-compulsive disorder, but psychodynamic psychotherapy is an ineffective treatment for the disorder. Neurobiology enriches our understanding of substance dependence, but psychopharmacology is *not* the mainstay of treatment for most substance-use disorders.

With these issues in mind, let's proceed with an admittedly brief, undoubtedly biased, tour of some of the theoretic perspectives you'll encounter.

GENETICS

A few diseases of 100% genetic origin have characteristic behavioral manifestations, such as the self-mutilation seen in Lesch-Nyhan syndrome. Other genetically based disorders, such as Huntington's disease, may manifest with a wide variety of psychiatric symptoms. When it comes to the idiopathic psychiatric disorders, however, the role of genetics becomes murkier, albeit of undeniable importance. (If it weren't murky, these disorders would no longer be idiopathic.) Of course, the importance of genetics varies from one disorder to another. In most disorders, the genetic influence is polygenic (multiple genes in the same individual or different loci in different individuals) and also multifactorial (i.e., the disorder is the result of a complex interplay between genetic factors and a variety of physiological, developmental, psychological, and social events). Some disorders may be largely genetic in origin (e.g., pervasive developmental disorder [autism], bipolar disorder). Some may be strongly genetic in some patients and less so in others (e.g., major depression). And for some disorders, genetic factors may play a more distant role or be predisposing but not causative (e.g., post-traumatic stress disorder and, perhaps, many personality disorders).

Researchers demonstrate genetic influences using a range of methodologies that include clinical (family or twin) studies and molecular biology techniques. As clinicians, though, we are forced to make crude guesses as to the contribution of genetics in a given patient, based on the family history along with what the larger research literature says about our patient's disorder.

NEUROBIOLOGY

Of course, the term "neurobiology" is so broad as to be largely meaningless by itself when used to refer to theories of psychopathology. It should be obvious that altered brain function is at least a concomitant of all altered behavior, although our current technology may or may not enable us to identify the brain dysfunction. Whether the altered brain function is a cause, a contributor, or an effect of the altered behavior is often the source of great debate and, undoubtedly, is quite different for different disorders. Also, our knowledge and technology are too crude for us to have a definitive lab test for the major idiopathic disorders. We can speak of neuroimaging abnormalities in, say, schizophrenia, but the diagnosis of schizophrenia remains a clinical one; a magnetic resonance imaging (MRI) scan will not rule in or rule out the diagnosis.

A wide array of techniques has been used to study neurobiologic abnormalities in psychiatric disorders. Neurochemically, most attention has focused on the "big three" neurotransmitters (dopamine, serotonin, and norepinephrine), with alterations noted in activity, neurotransmitter turnover, or receptor regulation for various disorders. Other neurotransmitters have been studied in relation to specific disorders or symptoms (e.g., cholinergic systems in Alzheimer's disease or gamma-aminobutyric acid [GABA] in anxiety disorders).

Neuroendocrine systems may also be altered in psychiatric disorders. The hypothalamic–pituitary–adrenal axis has been commonly studied, especially in relation to affective disorders and suicidal behavior. However, many other systems may be involved in particular disorders. For example, thyroid function and female reproductive hormones have been especially noted, if far from clearly understood, in their relation to psychopathology.

Psychoneuroimmunology is a relatively young field that posits the previously heretical notion that the brain and the immune system have the ability to talk to and influence each other. More specifically, behavioral events can affect, or be affected by, the state of the immune system. The relationships of these systems to specific psychopathologies remain speculative at this time, but are clearly a hot area for research in coming years.

Modern neuroimaging techniques are adding to our knowledge of brain correlates of psychiatric disorders. Early structural findings from computed tomography (CT) are now being revisited with MRI, which offers several advantages, including greater resolution of anatomic detail. Studies also have moved increasingly from crude assessments of overall brain atrophy or agenesis (as measured by total brain volume or ventricular–brain ratio) to examination of specific regions or structures (e.g., the dorsolateral prefrontal cortex in schizophrenia and the basal ganglia and frontal lobes in depression). Other techniques using molecules tagged with radioisotopes, such as positron emission tomography (PET) or single photon emission computed tomography (SPECT), hold promise for revealing functional neuroanatomy, a promise soon to be expanded by the use of echoplanar MRI. These various neuroimaging techniques have engendered well-deserved excitement in psychiatry. However, the diagnosis and management of most psychiatric disorders are clinically based. In day-to-day clinical work, there are no pathognomonic findings on neuroimaging scans other than the identification of more traditional neurological processes (e.g., neoplasms or vascular disease) that might contribute to psychiatric symptoms.

Neuropathology is at present even less useful than neuroimaging to most clinical psychiatric work. Brain biopsies are rarely conducted or indicated in psychiatric populations, and postmortem examinations of single cases are usually not illuminating. However, the concept of fine-level neuroanatomic abnormalities in major psychiatric disorders must not be dismissed, as was unfortunately done earlier in this century. For example, recent studies of schizophrenia have noted alterations in the organization of neuronal architecture in specific cerebral cortical layers.

Other investigative approaches shed light, to varying degrees, on brain function. Sleep architecture, as studied by electroencephalography (EEG) and measurements of systemic physiology, is altered in a number of psychiatric disorders—not just the primary sleep disorders but also mood disorders, chronic psychotic disorders such as schizophrenia, and others. Studies of chronobiology, including both seasonal and circadian (daily) biorhythms, are of increasing interest to those who wish to understand certain psychiatric disorders. Neuropsychological testing allows the examination of cognitive functions that may be tied to particular neuroanatomic regions or pathways, offering a complementary window on regional brain function.

PSYCHODYNAMICS

Psychodynamic concepts and theories dominated much of American psychiatry in the post–World War II era and to this day still dominate most laypersons' image of psychiatry, sometimes to pejorative effect. True, there were excesses during the heyday of psychoanalysis, both because other perspectives often were excluded from consideration and because some practitioners raised too high the expectations that psychodynamics would explain all mental disorders and lead directly to effective treatments for them. However, psychodynamic perspectives remain fundamental in understanding and working with the mentally ill. Psychodynamic thought has many permutations, but the following three concepts are basic to all else and will be useful not only in your psychiatry rotation but in your work with patients in all settings.

First is the notion of the *unconscious*. Simply put, much human mental activity—thoughts, feelings, conflicts, attempts at problem-solving—

happens outside of conscious awareness. At least some of this unconscious activity cannot be brought easily into awareness. Considerable human behavior that appears on the surface to be irrational or inexplicable may become understandable (though not necessarily reasonable or acceptable) if one can learn about the unconscious mental processes that underlie the behavior.

Second, you should become familiar with the range of what are termed *defense mechanisms*. In traditional psychoanalytic frameworks, defense mechanisms are unconscious mental acts that allow the individual to mediate ("deal with") unconscious intrapsychic conflicts, typically a conflict between wanting something and simultaneously recognizing that this want is unacceptable for some reason. Defense mechanisms come into play as a way out, a way to mediate the conflict. More broadly, and in more common use today, the term "defense mechanisms" refers to a wide range of problem-solving or coping skills, including those that happen quite consciously as well as those that occur unconsciously (Table 3–1). Defense mechanisms work, or otherwise we wouldn't use them. But some defenses work better than others. "Better" may mean more fully, that is, allowing a more successful resolution of the conflict or problem at hand. Or "better" may mean more flexibly in a variety of settings. Thus, persons with a more limited repertoire of defenses, or who rely on more "primitive" defenses, may be able to handle certain stressors well and yet not do well (e.g., develop troublesome psychiatric symptoms) under other circumstances. It is important for you during the clerkship to develop your ability to describe and assess patients' defenses. What defenses does your patient use most prominently? How well are the defenses working for your patient at this time? Understanding these issues is crucial to developing

Table 3–1. DEFENSE MECHANISMS (UNCONSCIOUS UNLESS OTHERWISE SPECIFIED)*

- *Denial*—awareness of external reality is kept out of consciousness. May reach delusional proportions *(psychotic denial)*.
- *Distortion*—as it says, distorting perception or recollection of external reality to meet defensive needs.
- *Projection*—unacceptable feelings or wishes are attributed to others. May reach psychotic proportions (e.g., persecutory delusions).
- *Projective identification*—a more complex defense mechanism that involves a relationship with another person, such as a psychotherapist. Unacceptable feelings or wishes are projected onto the therapist, and then behaviors are elicited from the therapist to confirm the projection. (For example, a patient with poor self-image might project this onto the therapist, with accompanied complaints that the therapist doesn't care about the patient. The patient then acts in such a fashion as to elicit anger or withdrawal by the therapist, thereby "confirming" the projection.)
- *Splitting*—other people are experienced as either wholly good or bad objects, with associated positive or negative affects. No gray zone exists. This may lead to swings between overidealizing and devaluing others, or to creating splits between "good guys" and "bad guys" (e.g., among a multidisciplinary treatment team).
- *Acting out*—unacceptable wishes are literally acted upon, but are not experienced consciously.
- *Passive-aggressive behavior*—aggression or rage expressed indirectly by inactions such as procrastination or "forgetting" a task.
- *Dissociation*—a substantial, if time-limited, alteration in one's consciousness, memory, or sense of personal identity.
- *Displacement*—shifting of affects from one object to another, e.g., after a long, frustrating day at work (with attendant anger at one's boss), coming home and yelling at one's spouse or kicking the cat.

Continued

Table 3–1. DEFENSE MECHANISMS (UNCONSCIOUS UNLESS OTHERWISE SPECIFIED)* *Continued*

- *Repression*—unconsciously mediated removal of an unacceptable impulse or affect from consciousness.
- *Externalization*—related to but broader than projection, involves perceiving one's own attributes and (more often) liabilities in the environment and other persons. Persons with prominent externalizing styles blame circumstances and other people rather than accepting responsibility for their own actions.
- *Reaction formation*—consciously experiencing an unacceptable wish or affect as its opposite.
- *Intellectualization*—using intellectual processes to minimize or avoid painful affects, impulses, or thoughts. Closely tied to *rationalization,* in which unacceptable behaviors, thoughts, or feelings are explained away as being reasonable.
- *Altruism*—constructively gratifying one's instincts by service to others.
- *Anticipation*—reality-based planning for, or worrying about, future inner discomfort.
- *Humor*—the constructive use of humor to manage difficult thoughts or affects.
- *Sublimation*—productively channeling instincts from socially unacceptable to acceptable or desirable ends.
- *Suppression*—consciously choosing or planning to postpone attention to a difficult impulse or affect.

---

*The earlier defenses in this list are more "primitive"; the later more flexibly adaptive.
(Adapted from Vaillant, GE: *Empirical Studies of Ego Mechanisms of Defense.* American Psychiatric Press, Inc., Washington, DC, 1986, pp 105–117, with permission.)

psychotherapeutic treatment plans, which may include helping patients to use existing defenses more effectively, to decrease the use of particularly dysfunctional defenses, or to develop a broader range of healthy defenses.

Finally, the notion of *transference* is crucial to understanding patient-physician relationships. Whenever we meet someone new, such as a doctor, we bring our own set of expectations, hopes, fears, and emotional reactions to the relationship. All this "baggage" is based on our own personalities and prior experiences and is, therefore, present before we even meet the new person. Also, much of this baggage is unconscious; that is, we may not be actually "thinking out loud" about our expectations or affects. Nonetheless, the baggage is real, and can profoundly affect the way we view the new person. When we actually meet and develop a relationship with our new physician, for instance, there is a complex interplay of our preexisting baggage with the external "reality" of the new physician, including his or her appearance, demeanor, and the subtleties of how the relationship forms and evolves.

This idea of transference may seem a bit too fancy or abstruse until you start to think of examples from your own clinical experiences. Perhaps some patients have distrusted you and your recommendations, while others have trusted you so completely that they were happy to follow your advice with little questioning or contemplation. That you could evoke such different responses, even though you were the same "you" with each patient, is evidence enough of the phenomenon of transference. How patients react to you will, in turn, affect how you interact with them, and so the doctor-patient relationship builds in varying directions, depending on the patient's transference, on those characteristics in yourself that are relatively immutable (age, gender, appearance, demeanor), *and* on how your own emotional response to the patient colors your interactions. This latter phenomenon, called *countertransference*, is essentially the transference of the physician toward the patient;

after all, physicians bring their own unconscious and conscious baggage to relationships just as everyone else does.

Why is transference so important? Well, during your psychiatry rotation, many of your patients will have particularly strong transference reactions that may make forming a treatment alliance difficult or stormy. You will also undoubtedly have your own strong countertransferences to many patients, given differences in life experiences, cultural backgrounds, or the behaviors and symptoms that led them to treatment in the first place. One of the goals of your clerkship should be to cultivate an educated awareness of these issues with two objectives:

1. To prevent your countertransferences from adversely affecting your interviews and alliance-building (which is very different from saying you shouldn't have reactions to your patients—we all do, and should)
2. To develop your skills at altering your interview style or approach in response to specific patient transference patterns, skills that will go a long way in helping you work effectively with a wide range of patients

BEHAVIORAL PSYCHOLOGY

Unlike psychodynamics, with its focus on intrapsychic processes, behaviorism focuses on external, directly observable behaviors. Much of what is known as behavioral therapy is rooted in learning theory with its notions that specific behaviors can be promoted or reduced by what are called *reinforcers*, that is, responses in the environment that encourage or discourage the behaviors. For example, an adolescent girl's suicide attempt may lead her family to rally in support. This natural, helpful response might, however, serve as a positive reinforcer for suicidal behavior. That is, the adolescent may learn that suicidal acts lead to increased family support, and thus suicidal behavior might increase in frequency. (Astute treating clinicians will recognize this potential and help the patient learn how to meet her needs without using suicidal acts.)

Clinicians use behavioral techniques with a variety of disorders and symptoms (see Chap. 15). All have in common ways of essentially encouraging (reinforcing) desired behaviors, and discouraging (extinguishing) dysfunctional or dangerous behaviors.

COGNITIVE PSYCHOLOGY

Cognitive psychology studies the way people think. As related to psychiatric disorders, it describes the characteristic ways in which people think while suffering from particular emotional states, such as depression or panic attacks. Cognitive psychologists would argue that these emotional states stem from problematic thinking and that dysfunctional patterns of thoughts often occur automatically and lead to the affective symptoms and other components of the disorder. These *cognitive distortions* may affect how one views oneself, the external environment, or the future. Examples of distortions include:

- *Dichotomous thinking*—perceiving things as either/or, black/white, good/bad, and so forth
- *Minimization and maximization*—selectively prioritizing the importance of certain facts, such as dwelling on one critical comment

made by a coworker while ignoring his or her many praising comments
- *Overgeneralization*—basing broad, sweeping beliefs on few or single incidents
- *Arbitrary inference*—coming to a belief or conclusion without direct evidence
- *Personalization*—taking events personally without evidence for such a connection
- *Selective abstraction*—dwelling on one small part of a more complex, larger situation

Understanding these ideas leads to cognitive psychotherapeutic approaches to treatment, in which patients learn to identify their dysfunctional thoughts and replace them with more functional, less distorted thoughts. In some ways, this approach is almost a behavioral therapy applied to internal thoughts, and often clinicians speak of using cognitive/behavioral techniques, as will be discussed further in Chapter 15.

GROUP PSYCHOLOGY

A number of psychological theories tackle the task of understanding human behavior in groups. The key tenet here is that groups manifest their own properties, affected by the properties of the individuals in the group, but also affected by group-level factors including the group's size, goals or tasks, and leadership. Group psychology is important to nonpsychiatric work such as psychological assessment of organizations (e.g., corporations). In psychiatric settings, theories of small-group dynamics underlie approaches to group psychotherapy, as discussed in Chapter 15.

FAMILY SYSTEMS

This perspective recognizes that families are complex systems that have their own characteristic patterns of interaction, both within the family and in relation to the rest of the world (including the physician). There is no single theory, of course, that explains all family interactions, but clinician encounters with families are guided by principles derived from several conceptual frameworks. Perhaps the most important fundamental concept is the importance of the relationship among individuals in a family and the family as a whole; one cannot understand the family without understanding the individuals, but behavior within the family takes on a complexity that must be evaluated at the level of the family and not solely as the sum of the individuals. Following from this, a patient presenting with psychiatric symptoms or disorders cannot be fully understood without appreciating his or her family in both its history and current state. Also, meetings with the family may be essential, not just for data-gathering purposes, but often to achieve successful psychotherapeutic ends.

DEVELOPMENTAL PERSPECTIVES

There is no single, catch-all developmental theory, of course. Human development occurs in a number of realms (including various physiological, psychological, and interpersonal factors) across the life span, and several theories may offer useful perspectives even about a "single" domain such as personality. Yet two broad perspectives are worth considering as you formulate each patient.

First, where is your patient *now* in his or her developmental course, and how successfully (or not) is he or she adapting to the demands of current developmental needs and challenges? For example, coping with physical or cognitive disability may have different meanings to a 40-year-old than to an 80-year-old, not that it is necessarily harder to cope at age 40, but the person's experience of his or her disability will differ based on the normal expectations of the patient and his or her peers. As another example, a college student's depression may be best understood by considering the student's experiences with negotiating the developmental tasks he or she faces, such as separation from family, establishing a sense of independent identity and efficacy, and so on.

Second, a developmental perspective may offer insights into current behavioral patterns as influenced by earlier life experiences. It's important not to oversimplify in this manner. Still, for example, it is a reasonable, educated speculation to postulate that a childhood of repeated abandonment by foster caregivers has contributed to a 20-year-old's current poor sense of self and tendency toward depressive symptoms and self-destructive acts.

OTHER PERSPECTIVES

Any list of perspectives relevant to understanding psychopathology must eventually come to an "other" category. Adherents of particular perspectives may be outraged to find their own pet viewpoint relegated to the dustbin of "other," or perhaps not mentioned at all. Yet the alternative is not to construct a list like this in the first place. Having begun, let us take a deep breath and try to finish the "unfinishable."

Again, a wide variety of additional vantage points are often useful. (I was going to say profitable, but, in these times, the use of that adverb seems ill-advised.)

- *Cultural* perspectives recognize the profound influence of culture on psychological and interpersonal processes and on the expression of and response to psychopathology.
- *Interpersonal* viewpoints obviously focus on the patient's interactions with others; here clinical attention may be used quite effectively, as exemplified by the use of interpersonal psychotherapy to treat major depression.
- *Couples* therapy draws on many family and interpersonal theories and focuses attention on the dynamics of a two-person system (dyad).
- *Ethics* is, of course, a perspective in all of medicine; psychiatry tends to highlight a number of issues, including those related to autonomy and consent.
- *Forensic psychiatry* includes legal aspects related to the usual care of psychiatric patients (including informed consent, confidentiality, and involuntary commitment to treatment—see Chap. 19), and also addresses the issues in which psychiatry and the criminal justice system come into contact (e.g., the relationship of mental disorder to criminal actions and competency to stand trial).
- *Community psychiatry* focuses attention on populations, including examining psychopathology from an epidemiological perspective. It also includes consideration of health services delivery: studying, modifying, or de-

signing systems of care for the large numbers of chronically disabled mentally ill persons who traditionally have depended on state or federal sources for treatment (e.g., state hospitals, community mental health centers, and Veterans Affairs hospitals).

2
PART

Psychopathology: The Basic Syndromes

"I got a head full of ideas that are driving me insane."
Bob Dylan, *Maggie's Farm,* 1965

"And my best friend, my doctor, won't tell me what it is I've got."
Bob Dylan, *Just Like Tom Thumb's Blues,* 1965

Bob Dylan's doctor friend obviously hadn't read this next section. These chapters provide a guided tour through the broad categories of psychiatric diagnoses. Some diagnoses will be covered in more depth than others, based on my admittedly idiosyncratic sense of what most trainees can and need to hear as they begin a psychiatry rotation.

4
CHAPTER

"Organic" Mental Disorders or Cognitive Disorders and Secondary Syndromes

Although the *Diagnostic and Statistical Manual of Mental Disorders* (DSM-IV) has adopted the phrase "cognitive disorders and secondary syndromes," the term "organic" has been used for a long time to describe mental disorders, and undoubtedly you will continue to hear it for some time to come. "Organic" is placed in quotes because brain dysfunction (however subtle or poorly understood) must be a concomitant, though not necessarily the "cause," of all psychiatric illness. In organic mental disorders, however, there are one or several known or presumed physical illnesses that directly affect brain function, which in turn directly leads to altered behavioral and symptomatic phenomena.

In Chapter 2, I pointed out that specific medical disorders may manifest as myriad psychiatric syndromes, and specific psychiatric syndromes may have many potential causes. It is also worth remembering that a psychiatric syndrome may be the first or even the only manifestation of a new medical or neurological process. Therefore, think differential diagnosis when evaluating a psychiatric presentation!

ETIOLOGY

The list of potential causes of psychiatric syndromes is long and, in fact, basically includes much of the rest of medicine. Rather than waste space with a useless list, what follows is a list of *types* of disorders to consider, organized in a way useful in psychiatry.

Intrinsic Central Nervous System Disease

It should make intuitive sense that disorders in this category, listed below, may lead to psychiatric symptoms since, by definition, they directly affect brain function:

- Congenital defects
- Toxins
- Tumors
- Cerebrovascular disorders (e.g., infarcts, hemorrhage, vasculitis)
- Infection (e.g., meningitis, encephalitis, human immunodeficiency virus [HIV], neurosyphilis)
- Demyelination
- Degeneration (e.g., Alzheimer's disease, Parkinson's disease)
- Hydrocephalus (e.g., obstructive, normal pressure hydrocephalus)
- Seizures (including auras and postictal and interictal states)

Systemic Diseases

It will be intuitively apparent that some of the following disorders can affect brain function (e.g., endocrinopathies), but others will not be so obvious. For example, why should bacterial cystitis, in the absence of bacteremia or sepsis, affect the brain? Yet it can, as can these others:

- Infection (from an isolated abscess or cystitis to full-blown sepsis)
- Cardiovascular/hematologic disorders (e.g., congestive heart failure, low-output states, anemia, hyperviscosity states)
- Metabolic disorders (e.g., hypoxemia, electrolyte disturbances, renal or hepatic failure, porphyria, burns, diabetes mellitus)
- Endocrine disorders (e.g., of the thyroid, adrenal cortex or medulla, sex hormones)
- Nutritional deficiencies (e.g., vitamin B_{12}, thiamine, niacin)
- Cancer

Drugs

Both recreational and medicinal preparations can cause psychiatric syndromes by either intoxication or withdrawal. *Intoxication,* in this context, means having the drug in one's system. It is important to note that medicines can cause psychiatric symptoms even if they are in the therapeutic range. For example, even when used appropriately, theophylline may cause anxiety, and glucocorticoids may induce mania. Also, some drugs, particularly drugs of abuse and psychotropic medications, are used intentionally to affect psychiatric symptoms. Thus, neuroleptics may be used to decrease psychotic symptoms, but they may also have the side effect of lowering the mood state. Similarly, cocaine may be injected to produce a euphoric mood state but may induce persecutory delusions.

Withdrawal refers to any state of reducing or eliminating a drug from one's system. Most commonly we think of withdrawal from recreational drugs, but some prescribed medicines may produce psychiatric withdrawal symptoms (e.g., anxiety from beta-blocker cessation).

The list of drugs associated with psychiatric symptoms is quite long, although the evidence for many of the associations is more anecdotal than carefully established. Some common offenders to keep in mind include:

- Drugs of recreational use, abuse, and dependence
- Psychotropics
- Anticholinergics
- Steroids (glucocorticoids and sex steroids)
- Histamine$_2$ blockers
- Many antiarrhythmics (e.g., digoxin, lidocaine)
- Beta-adrenergic blockers

PHENOMENOLOGIC TYPES

The organic mental disorders come in two basic flavors: the *secondary syndromes*, which by definition symptomatically resemble their idiopathic counterparts though they have an organic etiology, and the *cognitive disorders*, which, by virtue of having prominent cognitive deficits, are usually distinguishable from idiopathic psychiatric disorders.

The secondary syndromes are readily named according to their characteristic feature:

- Hallucinosis due to . . . (e.g., digoxin toxicity)
- Anxiety disorder due to . . .

- Delusional disorder due to . . .
- Mood disorder due to . . . (specify depressed, manic, etc.)
- Personality disorder due to . . .

The cognitive disorders can be broken down further into those with *global* cognitive deficits (more than one realm of cognition is affected) versus *mono*deficit disorders. *Amnestic disorder* is the term used for the single deficit of impaired memory. The two global cognitive disorders are *delirium* and *dementia,* which will be discussed in more depth in the following sections. In all cases, the etiology should be specified when known (e.g., dementia due to cerebrovascular disease).

DELIRIUM

Delirium can be defined as *transient fluctuating global cognitive dysfunction.* If you understand this sentence completely, you'll know more than most physicians do. Why is delirium important?

- Delirium has enormously high prevalence in medically ill populations such as those found on medical and surgical inpatient floors.
- Delirium is associated with increased rates of morbidity and mortality, for both the short term (e.g., in the hospital) and the long term.
- Delirium may be the first or most prominent manifestation of a change in the patient's physical status.

Therefore, *delirium should be regarded as a medical emergency until proven otherwise,* although for many patients it does turn out to have a nonemergent etiology. Yet, despite its importance, delirium is frequently missed or misdiagnosed. Why?

- A semantic muddle doesn't help. There are at least a couple of dozen synonyms in common use, such as "metabolic encephalopathy," "acute organic brain syndrome," and "acute confusional state." These varied terms tend to hamper clinicians from thinking of a common core psychiatric syndrome.

- Delirium is often multifactorial. A delirious patient may have a hematocrit of 32, a sodium level of 131, mild congestive heart failure, and an arterial oxygen saturation of 87%. Individually, these factors might not cause the delirium, but additively, they may. Beware of a clinician who claims that a patient can't be delirious because the "numbers" aren't bad enough.

- Similarly, beware of clinicians who claim the patient can't have delirium because there are *no* evident causes. If a patient has the clinical syndrome, then he or she has delirium. It's your job to determine why. You may or may not eventually figure this out, but your ignorance of the etiology shouldn't make you pretend the syndrome isn't there.

- Delirium can be quite varied in its clinical manifestations. The word "protean" is often used to describe this, and it's an accurate, if obscure, word to use. Besides its core features, which define the syndrome, delirium has a number of associated symptoms, which may in fact be more prominent than the core symptoms. The key is to identify the core syndrome and not be misled by the extra clinical stuff. So what are the core and extra features?

Core Features of Delirium

The core features of delirium are:

- Acute onset (typically hours to days, rather than weeks to months)
- Transiency (usually lasts days to several weeks, usually ends in complete resolution or death)
- Fluctuating course (Patients may look very different from one moment to the next: If you see wide variation, such as from lucidity one minute to complete disorientation the next, this is an excellent tip-off to delirium.)
- Altered level of consciousness (a key feature, since you don't see true lethargy or stupor as part of most idiopathic psychiatric disorders)
- Impaired attention (may be evident as distractibility or perseveration during conversation, not just on formal testing)
- Disorientation (Severe disorientation to place or time is again unusual in most idiopathic psychiatric disorders.)
- Other cognitive impairment (anything or everything—memory, language, praxis, visual-spatial impairment)
- Disorganized thinking (e.g., loosening of associations)

Other Common Features

Although the above are the core features of delirium, the following are also common:

- Mood disturbance (sad, euphoric, anxious, irritable)
- Psychosis (delusions, hallucinations, thought process derailments)
- Psychomotor changes (agitation, slowing)

- Disturbed sleep-wake cycle (from mild insomnia or hypersomnia to total loss of normal 24-hour rhythms)
- Neurological findings (subtle tremor, dysarthria, and gait ataxia)

Remember that these "extra" features may be more prominent than the core symptoms. Too many patients are referred for treatment of depression because they do in fact have a depressed mood and other depressive symptoms, but they turn out also to have the classic fluctuating course and cognitive deficits of delirium. Treatment implications are important here! For instance, giving antidepressants to a delirious patient will probably only worsen the delirium.

Assessment

How do you assess delirium? As always, begin with history, looking specifically for the time course, fluctuations, and cognitive deficits characteristic of the core syndrome. At the same time, a thorough medical history (including a detailed medication and drug history) will usually give strong clues as to the most likely causes of the delirium. The physical examination must be as comprehensive as the patient's clinical state allows, looking for any evidence of processes that might contribute to the delirium. The neurological examination is particularly important, not only to search for focal or specific CNS processes, but to identify the nonfocal stigmata mentioned above (i.e., tremor, dysarthria, and gait ataxia) that often accompany drug-induced or metabolic delirium. A careful mental status examination is obviously crucial (too often it is done only cursorily) and must include detailed cognitive assessment.

Having done all this, you will have established the presence of delirium and may or may not have a pretty good idea as to what's causing it. How far you go from here with laboratory work depends entirely on the clinical picture. For example, a young, previously healthy patient presents to you with a clear-cut delirium after a recent overdose of diazepam (Valium). He has no abnormalities on the physical examination other than dysarthria and gait unsteadiness. For this patient, you might choose to check few or even no laboratory values as part of the delirium workup (although you might wish to order tests as part of the workup for the overdose itself). At the other extreme, if you have no clues as to the etiology of a delirium after taking a thorough history and performing a physical examination, you will need to proceed with laboratory investigations immediately. You probably will begin with blood work—a complete blood count (CBC); a check of electrolyte levels, glucose, blood urea nitrogen (BUN), creatinine, liver enzymes, arterial partial pressure of oxygen (PaO_2) or oximetry saturation; a urinalysis; and a toxicology screen. If these tests fail to lead to an etiology, then aside from further blood work (e.g., an analysis of levels of thyroid-stimulating hormone [TSH], serum thyroxine [T4], vitamin B_{12}, folate, RPR, and a consideration of HIV testing), you will need to proceed with an electrocardiogram (ECG) and a chest X ray. If, after all this, you're still baffled (which is uncommon), you should obtain a neuroimaging study (computer tomographic [CT] scan is probably the most easily and rapidly available means), followed by lumbar puncture. Again, most delirious patients do not need such a mega-workup because the history, physical, and basic laboratory data usually suggest likely causes. But delirium should be evaluated as a medical/neurological emergency until proven otherwise.

It is worth mentioning here that an electroencephalogram (EEG) shows generalized slowing in most deliria (although alcohol withdrawal delirium presents with a characteristic fast-wave pattern). Unfortunately, generalized slowing is not specific for delirium, and the degree of slowing does not correlate well with the severity of the delirium, so an EEG is usually not helpful in establishing the diagnosis. On rare occasions, though, an EEG might help clarify the diagnosis, such as in delirium due to atonic (i.e., no gross motor activity) status epilepticus.

Treatment

How do you treat delirium? Far and away most important is treating the underlying conditions as much as possible. The other main principle is to avoid all central nervous system (CNS)–active drugs as much as you can. It may be tempting to give a hypnotic for sleep disturbance, but doing so runs a high risk of worsening or prolonging the delirium. If the patient's delirium is accompanied by life-threatening agitation (hitting caregivers, pulling out needed intravenous lines), and nonpharmacological approaches such as a calm and quiet milieu or restraints do not work sufficiently, low doses of high-potency neuroleptics such as haloperidol may reduce the psychomotor agitation without worsening the delirium.

DEMENTIA

Dementia is defined as a syndrome of global cognitive impairment, including memory disturbance but also including at least one other cognitive realm. Its onset is after childhood, which distinguishes it from mental retardation. The common conception of dementia is of a chronic progressive disease affecting the elderly, and indeed the most common causes of dementia are both progressive and more prevalent in old age. There are dementia syndromes that improve or resolve, however, and younger persons are not entirely free from risk of dementing disorders. Consider this a pitch to think about differential diagnosis when evaluating dementia; don't give up too soon and assume that the prognosis is hopeless.

Of course, many persons (especially in older age groups) have at least some degree of cognitive impairment, yet do not have dementia. What is enough impairment to qualify for the diagnosis? Simply put, the cognitive deficits must interfere with the patient's functional level to count as dementia. Knowledge of the person's previous functional level is often crucial here. For example, a highly educated and intelligent person, say, a PhD-level professor of linguistics, may have a mild dementing disorder and yet still be more intelligent—and intellectually functional—than much of the general population. Yet this person's deficits prevent the pursuit of his or her academic interests at the previous degree of skill, so this person has suffered a functional decline from baseline and qualifies to be considered demented.

As with delirium, associated psychiatric symptoms may be very prominent or troublesome. These may include:

- Personality change (an exaggeration of pre-morbid features, or onset of new features)
- Mood disturbance (depression, euphoria, anxiety, irritability)
- Psychosis (in Dr. Alzheimer's original case report, persecutory delusions were the patient's presenting symptom!)

- Sleep disturbance
- Other "nonspecific" behavioral disturbances (e.g., yelling, aggressivity, wandering)

Assessment

The assessment of dementia is similar in broad outline to that of delirium. Again, a careful history, physical (including neurological) examination, and mental status examination are usually sufficient to make the diagnosis of dementia and to suggest the most likely etiology. Most clinicians agree that it is reasonable, in newly presenting dementia, to check the battery of blood and urine tests cited above for delirium and to order an ECG and chest x ray. Unlike delirium, however, clear-cut dementia syndromes do not need to be considered a medical emergency in and of themselves (that is, unless something else from the evaluation suggests an emergency). To date there are no laboratory findings in wide clinical use that are pathognomonic for Alzheimer's disease, the most common cause of dementia. The clinical diagnosis of Alzheimer's disease, although usually accurate, must technically be considered "probable" until confirmed at autopsy.

Given this lack of pathognomonic laboratory findings, reasonable opinions may differ as to the usefulness and cost-effectiveness of routine neuroimaging studies in dementia. Certainly, any features in the clinical workup that are atypical for Alzheimer's disease, or that raise the possibility of more specific neurological processes, should lead to the appropriate neuroimaging scan (generally magnetic resonance imaging [MRI] or CT). Lumbar puncture and EEG are clearly not part of the routine evaluation of dementia and should be reserved for cases in which they are specifically indicated.

Treatment

Treatment of dementia differs from that of delirium because the most common causes of dementia, Alzheimer's disease and cerebrovascular disease, are not reversible. Risk factors for disease progression (e.g., hypertension, diabetes mellitus) should be managed aggressively. Other comorbid conditions that might contribute at least partially to dementia progression should also be treated aggressively. Often this involves the simplification of medication regimens, particularly trying to minimize use of CNS-active medications.

Even when nothing further can be done to treat the cause of the dementia, much may be offered to patients and their families. Mood, psychotic, or other behavioral symptoms often respond well to pharmacological therapy, nonpharmacological interventions such as behavioral therapies, or both. Supportive psychotherapies with the patient (in the earlier phases of the illness) and with the family are essential to help educate, support, and guide them through the complex and difficult affects and tasks associated with such devastating chronic illnesses. Often crucial to this work are education and guidance regarding use of appropriate social agencies and community resources (home health care, residential facilities) and attention to the financial and legal issues raised by patients' potential loss of competency to care or make decisions for themselves.

DISTINGUISHING DELIRIUM AND DEMENTIA

Delirium and dementia are both disorders of global cognitive impairment, but they have very different implications for prognosis and for the degree of urgency and depth with which they should be evaluated. Making matters more complicated, these disorders often coexist. Indeed, preexisting dementia is a risk factor for becoming delirious when faced with a new physiological insult, and many acutely ill delirious patients will be found to have an underlying dementia when the delirium clears. Thus, distinguishing between the two can at times be difficult, even for experienced clinicians. The following guidelines provide a starting point, but no broad postulates suffice for all situations:

- *Time Course:* Gradual and insidious onset over months or years makes delirium alone unlikely (but beware of delirium superimposed on dementia). Rapid onset is consistent with delirium, but does not rule out dementia from some causes, such as traumatic brain injury.
- *Fluctuations:* Large and rapid shifts in cognitive state or associated symptoms are highly suggestive of delirium.
- *Specific Cognitive Deficits:* Level of consciousness, attention, and orientation are affected early and severely in delirium but may be relatively preserved in mild or early dementias, in which memory, language, visual-spatial skills, praxis, and so on may be more prominently impaired.

5

CHAPTER

Mood Disorders

The "great divide" of mood disorders is the distinction between unipolar and bipolar illnesses. Both manifest episodes of depression, but bipolar illnesses are characterized by manic episodes. The importance of this distinction rests on evidence for different etiologies (based on epidemiological and family studies) and on implications for treatment.

MAJOR DEPRESSION

"There must be a cloud in my head—rain keeps falling from my eyes."
—Dee Clark, *Raindrops,* 1961

The word "depression" is, regrettably, terribly nonspecific. It can refer to a mood state (which, of course, may be normal, or may be found in a variety of psychopathological states), a clinical syndrome (e.g., a major depressive syndrome due to hypothyroidism), or a relatively specific disorder. So again, it's important to think about differential diagnosis when evaluating a patient with depressive symptoms.

Major depressive syndrome is defined as a minimum of 2 weeks of at least 5 symptoms from a specified list in the *Diagnostic and Statistical Manual of Mental Disorders* (DSM-IV). One of the symptoms must be either depressed mood or decreased interests. While DSM-IV simply lists the symptoms, it is useful for you to consider them in clusters of symptom types:

- Mood: dysphoria (obviously!), but also possible nonreactivity of mood, anxiety, irritability
- Ideational/psychological: feelings of worthlessness, guilt, helplessness, hopelessness; decreased interests; anhedonia; decreased subjective ability to concentrate; suicidal thoughts or behavior; ruminative thinking (tendency to dwell on the same depressive theme; often somatic/nihilistic themes predominate)
- Neurovegetative: sleep change (insomnia or hypersomnia); appetite and weight change (up or down); anergia; decreased libido; psychomotor change (agitation and/or retardation); diurnal variation (most commonly worse in the morning)
- Neuropsychological: decreased performance on cognitive testing, usually related to poor effort and attention; occasionally (especially in the elderly) more profound cognitive impairment, but generally distinguishable from that seen in degenerative dementias such as Alzheimer's disease
- Functional: social withdrawal; impaired performance at work, school, or other tasks; in severe cases, hygiene or other basic personal tasks may be affected

Important subtypes to consider include:

- Psychotic (presence of delusions/hallucinations)

- Melancholia (defined by specific symptoms, e.g., nonreactivity of mood, early morning awakening, severe weight loss, psychomotor changes, diurnal variation)
- Seasonal (onset and remissions of episodes at particular times of year, not in relation to obvious seasonal psychosocial stressors)

Some depressions manifest more heavily on the neurovegetative side and others more on the psychological side; yet all are "major depression" if they meet the "2 weeks, 5 symptoms" criteria.

Major depressive disorder is an idiopathic condition in which patients have one or more episodes of major depression. It is probably not a single illness but a group of conditions with similar manifestations but widely differing etiologies. Accordingly, theories of the pathogenesis of major depression span the biopsychosocial gamut, from the genetic and neurobiologic through a variety of psychological (including psychodynamic and cognitive) and psychosocial (e.g., family, cultural) theories.

Treatments shown to be effective in major depression include both specific forms of individual psychotherapy and somatic therapies (antidepressant medications or electroconvulsive therapy [ECT]). The psychotherapies with specifically demonstrated efficacy are cognitive and interpersonal therapy, discussed further in Chapter 15. Depressions with melancholia tend *not* to respond to psychotherapies alone, and hence require somatic therapies, whereas nonmelancholic depressions may respond to psychotherapies *or* somatic therapies. Psychotic depressions also require somatic therapies, specifically ECT or combinations of antidepressants and antipsychotic medications. Light therapy is effective as a primary or adjunctive treatment for seasonal depressions, particularly for milder, nonpsychotic forms.

BIPOLAR DISORDER

Bipolar disorder is also an idiopathic condition, but its causes are probably not as heterogeneous as those of unipolar depressions. Neurobiologic factors, including genetics, probably play predominant roles in the etiology of most or all cases. Psychological and social factors often are related to timing and triggering of acute episodes, however, and to the many issues that affect long-term outcome, including treatment compliance and alliance with caregivers.

Bipolar disorder is characterized by recurrent episodes of mania. Most patients also have major depressive episodes, although so-called "unipolar mania" has been noted. Episodes of depression resemble those seen in unipolar disorder, although bipolar patients' depressions are more likely to demonstrate:

- "Reversed neurovegetative signs," (i.e., hypersomnia, hyperphagia, weight gain)
- Psychosis (including prominent hallucinations or thought-process disturbance, seen more rarely in unipolar depression)
- Poor response to nonsomatic therapies alone

Mania, like major depression, is a syndrome that can be seen in a variety of clinical conditions, including secondary ("organic") mania, mania as part of delirium or dementia, and mania as part of schizoaffective disorder. Manic episodes consist of discrete periods of time during which the patient exhibits the following core symptoms:

- Elevated (euphoric), expansive, or irritable mood; labile affect
- Goal-directed hyperactivity (e.g., spending

sprees, sexual sprees, incessant letter writing or telephone calling)
- Psychomotor agitation (e.g., pacing, fidgeting, physical aggressivity)
- Inflated self-esteem (grandiosity)
- Decreased sleep need (quite different from the anguished insomnia of depression)
- Speech: rapid, increased in amount (logorrhea), loud, pressured
- Subjective sense of racing thoughts
- Objectively observed flight of ideas (which may worsen to frank loosening of associations or even total incoherence)
- Distractibility

During manic episodes, some patients may have simultaneous manic and depressive symptoms, a state known as "dysphoric mania" (or "bipolar disorder, mixed," to use DSM-IV language). In addition to thought-process disturbance, psychotic symptoms may also include hallucinations or delusions.

Bipolar disorder tends to run a chronic, intermittent course. Most patients can improve between episodes. With proper treatment, episodes can be reduced in severity and frequency. However, compliance is problematic for some patients, perhaps even more so than for many other chronic disorders. A few bipolar patients have a chronic, continuous course despite maximum treatment efforts, remaining almost continuously either depressed or manic, or continuously switching between the two poles (rapid cycling).

The mainstay of treatment is mood-stabilizing drug therapy. Antidepressants, antipsychotics, and anxiolytics are mostly reserved for treatment of acute exacerbations, although some patients may require long-term use of these agents. Individual or family psychotherapies are often crucial to forming and maintaining the treatment alliances within which compliance issues can be addressed. Psychotherapy also provides the framework for management of ongoing stressors or dysfunctional behavioral patterns that might precipitate or exacerbate the bipolar disorder.

OTHER MOOD-RELATED SYNDROMES

Hypomania: essentially mania without the drawbacks. In other words, a period of time marked by manic symptoms, but without substantial impairment in social or occupational dysfunction.

Bipolar II: as distinguished from regular bipolar disorder, which is also known as "bipolar I." Bipolar II is characterized by episodes of major depression and hypomania. Its genetics are probably distinct from those of both bipolar I and unipolar depression.

Cyclothymia: characterized by periods of hypomanic symptoms (which never quite fulfill the criteria for a full manic syndrome) and depressive symptoms (which never quite fulfill the criteria for major depressive syndrome). Cyclothymia may be hard to distinguish from the affective instability of some severe personality disorders. (Indeed, such distinctions may be illusory.)

Dysthymia: chronic (more than 2 years, and usually a lot longer than that) depressive symptoms. Must include at least three symptoms, but not enough for a full major depressive syndrome. *May* respond to pharmacological or other therapies, but the prognosis is generally guarded, not surprising for a disorder defined by chronicity. (As for any medical disorder, the best predictor of future chronicity is past chronicity.) Often such chronic depressive symptoms are tightly interwoven with what appears to be character pathology. Full major depressive episodes may occur on top of years of dysthymia, the so-called "double depression."

Adjustment Disorder with Depressed Mood: technically not a mood disorder because it's listed in DSM-IV with the other adjustment disorders. I list it here because it often comes up in the differential diagnosis of patients with depressive symptoms. Remember that stressful events are often associated with "real" major depression. If your patient has enough symptoms (5) for long enough (2 weeks), so that they fulfill the criteria for major depression, then he or she has major depression and not an adjustment disorder.

Bereavement: in a way, the ultimate example of an "adjustment" disorder. Full major depressive syndromes after the loss of a loved one are so common as to be called normal. Bereavement is therefore listed in DSM-IV only as a "V code" (i.e., not a mental disorder). However, major depression *is* diagnosed following the death of a loved one if the depressive syndrome is unusually severe (e.g., persistent suicidal ideation) or prolonged. Definitions of "severe" or "prolonged" are, of course, imprecise, and the whole border zone between bereavement and mood disorder is made even murkier by the high prevalence of prominent and disabling depressive symptoms in grieving patients even months or years after the loss.

6

CHAPTER

Psychotic Disorders

Psychotic symptoms, by definition, include hallucinations, delusions, and severe thought-process disturbances (e.g., thought blocking, loose associations). Psychotic symptoms may be seen in a wide variety of psychiatric .conditions, including dementia, delirium, mood disorders, and secondary ("organic") psychotic disorders. (This principle should sound familiar by now—as always, think differential diagnosis!) Psychotic disorders are idiopathic conditions that manifest with psychotic symptoms, that do not have prominent cognitive deficits (except as noted later), and that, with one exception (schizoaffective disorder), do not have prominent mood symptoms.

SCHIZOPHRENIA

Schizophrenia is the most common and important of the psychotic disorders, with prevalence and morbidity sufficient to make it a major public health problem. First things first, though: Contrary to popular (mis)usage, schizophrenia does *not* mean "split personality" in the sense of what is properly termed "multiple personality" (which itself was renamed "dissociative identity disorder" in the *Diagnostic and Statistical Manual of Mental Disorders* (DSM-IV) for those of you keeping score). If you're etymologically curious, the term *schizophrenia*, which in fact does derive from the Greek for "split mind," was coined in reference to the split between thoughts and affect sometimes seen in these patients.

In any case, the hallmark of schizophrenia is periods of acute psychotic symptoms (delusions, hallucinations, disorganized speech, or grossly disorganized or catatonic behavior). These episodes usually must include two or more such symptoms, although one symptom is enough to qualify if it involves either bizarre (i.e., nonplausible) delusions or specific types of auditory hallucinatory experiences.

Schizophrenic patients may also have what are called *negative symptoms,* which include affective flattening, poverty of speech, and avolition (lack of initiation of normal behaviors, such as grooming, dressing, seeking social interaction, or pursuing other goal-directed tasks). Also, the disorder must, by definition, cause social or occupational dysfunction and must last longer than 6 months, including any prodromal and residual symptoms. Prodromal and residual symptoms may include attenuated versions of psychotic symptoms or solely negative symptoms.

The course of schizophrenia is typically marked by periods of acute symptomatic exacerbations. Some patients may be largely symptom-free and quite functional between episodes, while many are more chronically symptomatic. Those patients with prominent and persistent negative symptoms tend to have more severe ongoing disability than those with mainly "positive" (i.e., psychotic) symptoms, which usually—though not always—respond better to acute treatments. Schizophrenia is often thought of as a progressive illness. This is something of an exaggeration, since many patients remain stable or improve symptomatically, functionally, or both over time. It is certainly true, however, that many patients do suffer a gradual or stepwise decline in functional ability. It is also true that, for most patients, schizophrenia is a chronic, typically lifelong illness.

As with most prominent idiopathic psychiatric disorders, theories of etiology and pathogenesis run the full biopsychosocial gamut. The most prominent current notions emphasize the role of neurobiology, probably a combination of genetic and prenatal, perinatal, or early childhood-acquired factors. It is also quite clear that acute clinical exacerbations can be related to stressful events and circumstances.

As with other disorders, comorbidity substantially affects treatment and prognosis for schizophrenia. Substance dependence is a common comorbidity, which may directly add to the patient's psychotic symptoms (e.g., cocaine-induced delusional disorder). Such so-called "dual diagnosis" or "MICA" (Mentally Ill Chemical Abuser) patients need treatment different from that often provided in traditional psychiatric or substance-dependence treatment settings, and an increasing array of outpatient and inpatient services is developing in many communities to serve the specific needs of MICA patients.

In pursuit of the syndromic differential diagnosis of schizophrenia, evaluation must confirm that the phenomenology of the psychosis is not more consistent with that of another psychotic disorder (e.g., a sole symptom of monothematic nonbizarre delusions is more consistent with delusional disorder). The presence of prominent mood symptoms should raise the possibility of schizoaffective disorder or a primary mood disorder. Prominent cognitive deficits should raise questions about underlying, or even primary, mental retardation or dementia, although this may be difficult to assess in an acutely disorganized patient. (Also, in residual stages of schizophrenia itself, subtle deficits may be found in areas such as frontal executive functions.) Secondary causes of psychosis must be sought. This search often entails a neuroimaging study such as magnetic resonance imaging (MRI) in new-onset cases. Remember, though, that the fundamentals remain, well, fundamental (i.e., careful medical history, physical examination including neurological exam, and basic laboratory tests are essential). DSM-IV describes subtypes of schizophrenia based on the predominance of particular symptoms (e.g., paranoid, disorganized), although the prognostic utility of these subtypes is limited.

Psychotropic drugs clearly reduce the frequency and severity of acute symptomatic exacerbations and improve the quality of life for most people with schizophrenia. Traditional neuroleptics remain the mainstay for many patients, but newer atypical antipsychotics such as clozapine and risperidone help many who did not respond to or tolerate the older agents. Other drug classes may play adjunctive roles in acute circumstances (e.g., benzodiazepines) and less acute events (e.g., mood stabilizers). Electroconvulsive therapy (ECT) may be effectively used for intractable acute psychosis or associated mood-related symptoms such as suicidal ideation.

Most experts in the field would now agree that insight-oriented psychotherapy does not alter the basic psychopathogenesis of schizophrenia. Still, psychotherapies of various types play crucial roles in the management of this often chronic and debilitating disorder. Individual and group work usually focuses on psychoeducation (including expectations regarding disease course and the need for compliance with medications and follow-up treatment) and support (helping minimize the demoralization that may accompany profound disability). Many patients need guidance with the practical management of their day-to-day affairs, which may be provided by therapists, case managers, and group settings including social programs aimed at persons with similar needs. Families also often benefit from supportive and psychoeducational therapies. In fact, psychoeducational approaches with families lead to decreased expression of anger and hostility within the family, which decreases relapse rates in schizophrenic patients.

SCHIZOPHRENIFORM DISORDER

Patients with schizophreniform disorder manifest the same acute symptoms as do persons with schizophrenia, but the total duration of all symptoms and functional impairment is only 1 to 6 months. Some of these persons go on to a subsequent psychotic relapse, necessitating a change in diagnosis to schizophrenia. This diagnostic category recognizes that some patients' psychoses are time-limited.

SCHIZOAFFECTIVE DISORDER

As has been noted, most of the major psychiatric disorders are probably not single illnesses but rather phenomenologically similar-appearing conditions that we do not yet know how to distinguish from one another. Well, this caveat applies in spades to schizoaffective disorder, which is probably a heterogeneous grab bag of presen-

tations in the nebulous territory between schizophrenia and mood disorders. Indeed, an older research diagnostic scheme used the categories
"schizoaffective, mainly schizophrenic" and
"schizoaffective, mainly bipolar." These are terribly unwieldy terms for everyday clinical use; yet
they are instructive. It may well be that some
persons with schizoaffective disorder really have
schizophrenia (but with more prominent mood
symptoms than most), while others really have a
bad mood disorder (with more prominent psychotic symptoms than most).

To define this messy territory, DSM-IV criteria
for schizoaffective disorder stipulate that the patient must have periods of psychosis *without*
prominent mood symptoms *and* periods of full
mood syndrome (manic or major depressive)
concurrent with acute schizophrenic-type psychotic symptoms. Subtypes denote whether the
mood symptoms are depressive only or include
periods of mania (bipolar type).

Treatments for schizoaffective disorder, not
surprisingly, resemble the treatments for schizophrenia and mood disorders. Prognosis is quite
variable, although as a general rule the course of
illness is better when mood symptoms are more
prominent and psychotic symptoms less so.

DELUSIONAL DISORDER

In this disorder, stunning in the aptness of its
name, the characteristic feature is indeed delusions. To be specific, nonbizarre (that is, potentially plausible) delusions must be present for at
least 1 month. Thought-process disorganization
is *not* found, and hallucinations are either nonexistent or not prominent (although tactile or ol-

factory hallucinations may be prominent if they are directly tied to the delusional theme). In other words, the acute positive symptom criteria for schizophrenia are *not* met. Also, behavior and functioning are *not* impaired except as directly related to the delusional material. Thus there are no equivalents to the negative symptoms of schizophrenia. Several subtypes of delusional disorder are described, based on the predominant delusional theme: erotomanic, grandiose, jealous, persecutory, somatic, and the usual catchalls, mixed and unspecified.

Persons with delusional disorder come to psychiatric attention rather uncommonly. This is so because of their relative intactness of functioning, as well as their lack of insight into their illness. Only occasionally do their actions lead to the type of difficulties that cause others to force them to seek clinical care.

Etiology is, of course, unknown; if it were known, the diagnosis would change to that of a secondary disorder (e.g., cocaine-induced delusional disorder). Neurobiologic factors, while probably implicated, have received considerably less study than they have in schizophrenia or the major mood disorders. Many psychodynamic theories have focused on the delusions' defensive usefulness, as well as on their symbolic meanings. The course may often be chronic, although some degree of waxing and waning may occur. A few patients may have complete remissions, whereas others may become increasingly preoccupied with their delusional system.

Treatment involves maintaining a therapeutic alliance, no small task with patients who by the nature of their disorder lack insight and tend to externalize rather than openly discuss their internal world. If compliance can be achieved, neuroleptic drugs appear to help by reducing the intensity of the delusional preoccupation, even if they do not eliminate the psychosis entirely.

BRIEF PSYCHOTIC DISORDER

A catchall rather than a specific entity, this diagnostic term is used to classify any brief (i.e., over and done with in less than 1 month) episode of one or more psychotic symptoms. If associated with marked psychosocial stressors, this disorder corresponds to an older and still commonly used term, "brief reactive psychosis."

SHARED PSYCHOTIC DISORDER

This disorder is better known as *folie à deux* (French, more or less, for "crazies of two"). The patient with shared psychotic disorder comes to share the delusions of another person (someone who has a psychotic disorder, usually schizophrenia). Most often the patient has a close, live-in relationship with this other person. This disorder raises interesting questions about the relationships between environment and intrinsic diathesis (predisposition) toward psychosis. The disorder is rather uncommon and is treated with psychotropic medications and appropriate psychotherapeutic modalities.

7

CHAPTER

Anxiety Disorders

Anxiety is obviously a hallmark symptom of each of the disorders in this category. It is important to remember, though, that anxiety may be prominent in other "non-anxiety" disorders, including delirium, dementia, mood disorders (especially depression), and psychotic illnesses. Also, secondary anxiety disorders (due to general medical conditions or substance-induced) may demonstrate the clinical features of generalized anxiety, panic attacks, or obsessions and compulsions.

It is also useful to remember that anxiety—from any cause—is often associated with one or more somatic symptoms. These symptoms may involve virtually every organ system and anatomic region. A partial list of anxiety-associated symptoms is provided in Table 7–1.

PANIC DISORDER

Panic disorder is characterized by recurrent, unexpected, idiopathic panic attacks. These are followed by at least 1 month of worry about having another attack or about its consequences, or

Table 7–1. PHYSICAL SYMPTOMS THAT MAY BE ASSOCIATED WITH ANXIETY

Cardiopulmonary
Chest pain
Dyspnea
Tachycardia
Palpitations
Elevated blood pressure

Autonomic
Diaphoresis
Flushing
Hot flashes or cold spells
Dry mouth
Pupillary mydriasis

Gastrointestinal
Nausea or vomiting
Diarrhea
Abdominal cramping or other pain
Sense of dysphagia, choking, or "lump in the throat"

Neurological
Blurry vision
Paresthesias (perioral, extremities)
Tremor
Dizziness or lightheadedness
Muscle aches
Gait unsteadiness

Genitourinary
Urinary urgency, frequency, or hesitancy

by a change in behavior related to the attacks (e.g., avoiding certain places for fear of having another attack). Panic disorder may occur without or with agoraphobia.

So presumably you're now asking: What are panic attacks and agoraphobia? Patients often use the term "panic attack" indiscriminately to refer to any severe anxiety symptoms. A *true panic attack* occurs over a discrete period of time, typically for a few minutes to a few hours at the most. During this period, anxiety and at least four somatic symptoms (chosen from a list in the *Diagnostic and Statistical Manual of Mental Disorders* [DSM-IV] but all familiar to you from Table 7–1) develop and increase rapidly to a peak within 10 minutes. The panic attacks in panic disorder are special in that

- They are unexpected; that is, they don't always occur in predictable response to a particular situation. (If they do, see the section on phobias.)
- They are recurrent.
- They are idiopathic, that is, not drug-induced or due to a general medical condition.

Agoraphobia involves anxiety about circumstances in which the patient feels that escape is difficult or help is unavailable. Typical circumstances include being alone outside one's home, such as being alone in a crowd, on bridges, or in cars, buses, trains, and so on. (If the fears are limited to one specific situation, refer to the section on phobias below.) The patient avoids these situations, endures them with considerable distress and fear of having a panic attack, or demands to be accompanied. Just to confuse the uninitiated (and sometimes the initiated, too), agoraphobia may be part of panic disorder (as in "panic disorder with agoraphobia"), or may exist alone (cleverly termed "agoraphobia without history of panic disorder").

Panic disorder is rather common. It is more prevalent in women. Many patients presenting to general medical settings with specific somatic complaints (e.g., young women visiting emergency rooms with chest pain) have panic disorder. More data are needed regarding the naturalistic course (as opposed to studying just those patients who present for treatment). It is clear that with treatment most patients will do well, but in some (perhaps most), panic disorder will have a chronic course, especially if maintenance treatments are discontinued.

Pathogenetic theories for panic disorder run the usual biopsychosocial gamut and in their broad outlines are similar to those for most of the anxiety disorders. In early psychodynamic traditions, anxiety is a hallmark of unresolved unconscious conflict. More recent psychodynamic schools of thought, such as those built around object-relations theory, emphasize that proneness to unpleasant affects and fears results from the lack of a whole, internal sense of self and, thus, the lack of ability to soothe oneself without direct support from other people. (See more on this subject in Chap. 9.)

Treatments for panic disorder, supported by considerable and growing empirical research, have focused on cognitive/behavioral and neurobiologic models of the disorder. In cognitive psychological terms, panic attacks result from catastrophic misinterpretations of normal bodily sensations. These misinterpretations lead to anxiety, which in turn may amplify somatic symptoms, which then raises the anxiety level further, and so on in a vicious circle. Avoidant and agoraphobic symptoms are seen as a behavioral consequence of experiencing panic attacks and attempting to respond to what one has "learned" by avoiding situations that may provoke attacks. In this conceptual framework, psychotherapy focuses at first on the misinterpretations of somatic symptoms and helps the patient break the vicious circle by substituting more rational, hopeful interpretations, which, in turn, are accompanied by a reduction in anxious affect. After panic attacks are reduced or eliminated, behavioral psychotherapeutic approaches are used to help the patient reengage with previously avoided situations, so he or she can learn that such situations are now safe and will not necessarily lead to an unmanageable panic attack.

Neurobiologic theories have focused on what may be viewed as the inappropriate or excessive activation of the brain mediators of the "fight or flight" response. Multiple neurotransmitter systems are likely involved, including serotonin, gamma-aminobutyric acid (GABA), and various neuropeptides, but norepinephrine and its complex connections emanating from the locus coeruleus have received the most attention to date. From this perspective, treatment must dampen relevant neurobiologic systems to reduce panic attacks. Empirically effective medications include several antidepressants and fairly large doses of high-potency benzodiazepines such as alprazolam or lorazepam. Of course, successful psychotherapy may also work by ultimately dampening hypersensitive or hyperactive neurobiologic systems. In reality, most patients are probably treated with a combination of medications and a tailored blend of supportive, psychoeducational, and cognitive/behavioral psychotherapy.

PHOBIAS

Phobias are among the most common of mental disorders. They vary in severity and consequence from the relatively untroubling to the entirely disabling. The two main brands are specific (or simple) phobias, and social phobia. *Specific phobias* are, not surprisingly, fears of well-defined objects or situations (e.g., airplanes, heights, dogs). The attendant fear, or avoidance phenomena, must cause significant distress or affect the person's functioning or life routine. *Social phobias* involve distressing or disabling fears of social or performance situations, in which the patient is afraid that scrutiny or evaluation by others will lead to embarrassment or humiliation. Social phobias may themselves be circumscribed (e.g., a musician's "stage fright") or generalized to most social situations (in which case the additional diagnosis of *avoidant personality disorder* should be considered).

The main treatment of specific phobias is behaviorally based: Typically, the patient is gradually exposed to a series of situations that increasingly mimic his or her feared stimulus *(systematic desensitization)*. For generalized social phobia, cognitive/behavioral approaches (including desensitization and relaxation techniques) may be of some value, but pharmacotherapy (including monoamine oxidase inhibitors) has growing empirical support. Performance anxiety (stage fright) may respond to these measures; beta-adrenergic blockers, when taken prior to performance, may also help, probably by reducing sympathetically mediated anxiety symptoms such as tremor and palpitations.

OBSESSIVE-COMPULSIVE DISORDER

Let's start with what obsessive-compulsive disorder (OCD) is *not*. We all tend to think of "obsessive" as meaning rigidly preoccupied with details, often to the point of "not seeing the forest for the trees." And to "obsess" about something means to be preoccupied with worry about that subject. Well, these definitions are accurate in and of themselves, as applied to obsessive-compulsive personality disorder, discussed further in Chapter 9. However, OCD refers to much more specific symptoms, and OCD may or may not occur in relation to obsessive-compulsive personality style or disorder.

So what is OCD? Persons with OCD suffer from either obsessions or compulsions and often from both. To qualify as OCD, the obsessions and compulsions must cause significant distress, take up considerable time (more than 1 hour a day), or impair functioning.

Obsessions are defined as recurrent mental activity, which may be thoughts, impulses, or images. At some point the patient experiences these as intrusive or inappropriate, so-called "ego-alien" (e.g., "I know these thoughts make no sense, but they keep popping up in my mind."), although many OCD patients lose the ego-alien quality of their obsessions over time. In addition, to qualify as obsessions, the thoughts, impulses, or images:

- Must not be simply worries about actual, real-life problems
- Must not be solely the product of psychosis (e.g., delusions)
- Must be the focus of efforts by the patient to "get rid" of them somehow, often by attempts at distraction or suppression

Typical obsessions include themes of contamination, doubts about past actions, a need for order or symmetry, and aggressive or sexual impulses, thoughts, or images. Often patients describe a cycle wherein these annoying, ego-alien thoughts intrude on the mind, followed by attempts at suppression, which leads to mounting anxiety, until finally they abandon the suppressive efforts, with consequent relief of anxiety but recurrence of the unwanted obsession.

Compulsions are in some sense the equivalent

of an obsession in action. They are defined as repetitive behaviors (e.g., washing hands) or mental actions (e.g., counting). The patient feels driven to perform compulsive actions according to the dictates of an obsession or some rigid, self-imposed rules. Attempts to suppress the compulsion lead to mounting anxiety. As occurs with the ego-alien quality of obsessions, the patient recognizes that the compulsions are unreasonable or excessive at some point during the illness (although this may not be true for children).

Recent research has demonstrated that OCD is more common than previously thought, with a point prevalence of about 1.5%. Its course tends to be chronic, and many persons with more severe forms of OCD are quite incapacitated by their symptoms.

Psychodynamic perspectives have had a long-standing field day with OCD, paying attention to the symbolic meaning of the individual patient's specific obsessions and compulsions as unconscious mechanisms to manage what would otherwise be intolerable levels of anxiety. Such perspectives often lead to a rich understanding of the patient's mental life. However, psychodynamically based psychotherapies have not proven effective in reducing obsessions or compulsions.

Converging lines of evidence have suggested genetic and neurobiologic bases for OCD. OCD is probably related to tic syndromes such as Tourette's disorder. Dysfunctional brain regions may include the basal ganglia and frontal lobes. The mainstays of pharmacotherapy for OCD are serotonin-specific reuptake inhibitors (SSRIs). Their effectiveness has sparked interest in serotonergic-mediated disease mechanisms, but other neurotransmitter systems are probably also affected. Other pharmacological agents, alone or as adjuncts—including monoamine oxidase inhibitors, lithium, antipsychotics, and anxiolytics—may be helpful in the management of specific cases. In addition, behavioral therapies reduce the frequency of the symptoms, particularly compulsive rituals. Cognitive-behavioral approaches using individual, group, or family modalities are essential parts of the comprehensive treatment of OCD patients. In recent years, small studies suggest the effectiveness of limited psychosurgery (e.g., stereotactically guided cingulotomy) for severe and refractory OCD patients. For the foreseeable future, however, psychosurgery is likely to remain a treatment of last resort, used only for patients with severe OCD, because of the limited data on its use and the stigma that surrounds the alleged and actual abuses of more global psychosurgery ("frontal lobotomy") earlier this century.

POST-TRAUMATIC STRESS DISORDER

Post-traumatic stress disorder (PTSD) is a syndrome that arises in response to a psychologically traumatic event. The event must be of greater magnitude than the stressors most persons encounter frequently. DSM-IV defines the event as one that threatens death or serious physical harm to self or others and that produces intense feelings of horror, fear, or helplessness. Not all persons exposed to such events—be they victims of rape, physical assault, warfare, or natural disaster—develop PTSD, however. Some develop PTSD, some have depression, some develop other disorders (including anxiety, mood, and psychotic disorders), and some do not develop enough symptoms to warrant diagnosis of a mental disorder at all. In other words, as in most or all psychopathology, there is an interplay between external circumstances and a person's diathesis toward particular symptoms. Still, in PTSD the proximate cause of the disorder is the traumatic event: Without the event, the person wouldn't have PTSD.

To qualify for a diagnosis of PTSD, the patient must have symptoms in each of three realms:

- "Positive" or "re-experiencing" symptoms, including recurrent and intrusive memories of the event, dreams, event re-enactments (which may include hallucinations or full-fledged flashback episodes), and worsening distress when exposed to stimuli that resemble the event in some way
- "Negative" symptoms, including both avoidance (e.g., avoiding thoughts or discussions related to the event; avoiding persons, activities, or places that are reminiscent of the traumatic event; amnesia for part of the event) and numbing phenomena (e.g., decreased interests, feeling detached from others, affective flattening, or a sense of a foreshortened future)
- Symptoms of increased arousal, such as insomnia, irritability, trouble concentrating, hypervigilance, or exaggerated startle response

If a limited but specified array of the above symptoms is present for 2 days to 1 month after the traumatic event, DSM-IV assigns a diagnosis called *acute stress disorder*. PTSD is diagnosed if a larger array of symptoms is present for more than 1 month; subtypes include *acute* (up to 3 months), *chronic* (longer than 3 months), and *with delayed onset* (onset of symptoms more than 6 months after the event).

Only the positive, or reexperiencing, symptoms are unique to PTSD. Avoidance and hyperarousal symptoms may be seen in other anxiety disorders, as well as in mood disorders. Indeed, the course of PTSD may be complicated by the development of full-fledged major depression or other disorders, and comorbid diagnoses should be given and treated as appropriate.

Psychological theories of the pathogenesis of PTSD have used psychodynamic or cognitive frameworks to consider PTSD symptoms as resulting from attempts to cope with the unmanageable affects and thoughts arising from the traumatic event. Behavioral psychological perspectives consider PTSD symptoms as learned responses to cues associated with the original trauma. A growing range of investigations points to brain and neuroendocrine functional abnormalities, which presumably are caused by the psychological trauma. For example, altered central and peripheral noradrenergic function is present and may be part of what mediates the hyperarousal symptoms in PTSD.

Treatments for PTSD may profitably employ several modalities. An empathic relationship with an individual psychotherapist allows for exploration of the thoughts, images, and affects associated with the traumatic event. Such work is the mainstay of treatment shortly after the event happens (e.g., in acute stress disorder), although anxiolytics also may be useful in the short term. These psychotherapeutic techniques are also helpful in more chronic cases, both in and of themselves and to establish a treatment alliance within which behavioral or pharmacological treatments may be used. Behavioral techniques may include relaxation training and exposure methods designed to reduce the degree of symptoms caused by cues associated with the trauma. Medications should be used aggressively as indicated by comorbid syndromes such as depression. In addition, several classes of antidepressants, including tricyclics and monoamine oxidase inhibitors, may help with the positive and hyperarousal symptoms of PTSD itself. Other agents, including mood stabilizers, have been tried, but clear treatment guidelines for their use do not yet exist. Finally, group psychotherapies for patients exposed to similar traumatic events can be of great help, both acutely and in more chronic variants of the disorder.

GENERALIZED ANXIETY DISORDER

Basically, generalized anxiety disorder (or GAD, as it's called by those in the know) is a relatively grab-bag category of patients with anxiety symptoms that don't quite fit any other anxiety- or mood-disorder diagnosis. To qualify, the patient must have more than 6 months of excessive anxiety or worry, with at least 3 associated physical symptoms, to a degree that causes significant distress or dysfunction. A large part of the evaluation of such patients involves establishing that, in fact, the anxiety is not better explained by a secondary anxiety disorder or by some other idiopathic syndrome (e.g., panic attacks? obsessions? depressive symptoms?). GAD may be the most common of all the anxiety disorders, and it often runs a chronic course. Thus, it is commonly encountered in virtually all nonpsychiatric clinical settings.

Once the diagnosis is established, both psychotherapeutic and pharmacological treatments should be considered. A full continuum of psychodynamic psychotherapy may be useful—from expressive (addressing more fundamental intrapsychic needs and conflicts) to supportive (emphasizing the empathic alliance and stress-management approaches). Where along this continuum the therapy should fall at any given time depends on a variety of factors, including the patient's personality style, strengths, and vulnerabilities (including personality pathology); his or her capacity to form an interpersonal alliance with the therapist; the degree of symptomatology at the time; and the nature of the therapeutic setting (e.g., short- vs. long-term, frequency of visits). Cognitive and behavioral techniques are often useful too, paralleling their use in panic disorder. In terms of medications, benzodiazepines and buspirone are the mainstays. Clearly, the benefits and risks of their use (particularly of the benzodiazepines, with their addictive potential) must be weighed, but many patients will be legitimately helped by long-term use of these drugs. There may be a role for antidepressants as well, perhaps especially including the tricyclics, although their efficacy in GAD independent of panic attacks and depressive symptoms is not clear.

8

CHAPTER

Substance Use Disorders

"You know Canned Heat* is killing me."
— **Tommy Johnson,** *Canned Heat Blues,* 1928

The history, sociology, economics, pharmacology, and other aspects of substance-use disorders have made many a fine book and are well beyond the scope of this one. Suffice it to say that in the U.S. today, substance-use disorders are the most prevalent of all mental disorders, with enormous consequences for our population's mental and physical health and with tremendous consequences affecting society as a whole. No physician will escape encountering the myriad effects of substance-use disorders on patients and their families and communities.

---

* Canned Heat is a heating fuel, akin to Sterno, that contains ethanol, methanol, and acetone. Despite its toxicity, it was a relatively popular drink among alcoholics during Prohibition.

CONCEPTS AND DEFINITIONS

The *Diagnostic and Statistical Manual of Mental Disorders* (DSM-IV) classification of "substance-related disorders" can seem confusing. The following concepts should make it all—at least in principle—pretty straightforward.

Each substance class is listed separately:

- Alchohol
- Amphetamines
- Caffeine
- Cannabis
- Cocaine
- Hallucinogens
- Inhalants
- Nicotine
- Opioids
- Phencyclidine
- Sedative/hypnotic/anxiolytics
- Polysubstance (for the "bet you can't try just one" crowd)
- Other/unknown (for the truly unusual, or the commonplace scenario of clinician uncertainty)

Under each substance class you will find several possible types of disorders:

- Intoxications, which are substance-specific, reversible, maladaptive behavioral states caused by having the drug on board
- Withdrawal states, which are substance-specific maladaptive conditions caused by the reduction or cessation of intake of a substance
- Delirium syndromes due to intoxication or withdrawal involving a specific substance (e.g., alcohol withdrawal delirium)
- Specific mental syndromes caused by the substance, called substance-induced disor-

ders, resembling secondary syndromes (e.g., substance-induced psychotic, mood, anxiety, or sleep disorders, sexual dysfunctions, and dementias)

Finally, some disorders relate to the pattern of misuse of the substance. Although it is possible to have a substance-induced mental disorder, or a state of intoxication, *without* having a history of abuse (from, say, unlucky one-time use), most patients presenting with an intoxication or other substance-induced disorder have underlying troubles with recurrent substance use; these are termed *substance-use disorders*. (Withdrawal is another matter, of course, as we shall see.)

SUBSTANCE DEPENDENCE VS. ABUSE

DSM-IV defines two kinds of substance-use syndromes, *substance dependence* and *substance abuse*. In the real world, though, which includes a goodly portion of psychiatric settings as well as virtually all nonpsychiatric clinical settings, most people use the terms "dependence" and "abuse" more or less interchangeably.

To diagnose *substance dependence*, at least three of the following physiological and behavioral phenomena must occur within a 12-month period:

- Tolerance (more drug is needed to obtain the same effect)
- Withdrawal (use of more substance than planned, or over a longer time period than planned)
- Attempts to cut down or somehow modify the substance use pattern

- Much time spent in getting, using, or recovering from the substance
- Reduction of the time spent in other, non–substance-related activities
- Continued substance use despite the patient's knowledge of adverse consequences (which may range from depression to marital conflict to physical sequelae such as alcohol-associated gastritis)

Physiological dependence alone is not sufficient to be diagnosed with the mental disorder "substance dependence." For example, *any* patient who is prescribed opioids at a fixed dose for long enough will develop drug tolerance and will withdraw if the opioid is stopped suddenly: Such effects are built into the pharmacology of the drug. But if the patient takes the drug only as prescribed, and the drug intake does not adversely affect the patient's life (indeed, one would hope it would not be prescribed if it didn't *help*), then the patient does not suffer from a substance-use disorder.

Substance abuse is a lesser, but still potentially devastating, use disorder involving an adverse psychological or social consequence related to the substance use. It is lesser only because the diagnosis is not given if criteria for dependence are met (otherwise most patients with dependence would also be given a comorbid diagnosis of abuse, thus making the diagnostic muddle even more muddled). Adverse consequences might include:

- Impairment in performance at work or home
- Use in hazardous situations (e.g., driving while intoxicated)
- Legal problems related to substance use
- Continued use despite adverse effects on interpersonal relationships

ETIOLOGY

It's difficult to think about the causes of substance-use disorders *in toto*, because although many principles apply broadly, many factors are unique to specific drugs. Here we can only suggest the breadth of factors that need to be considered. Genetics clearly plays a role in some addictions, particularly alcoholism. Neuropharmacology mediates some of the reinforcing qualities of intoxication (e.g., the pleasurable high of cocaine) and withdrawal states (which, if unpleasant enough, will reinforce continued drug use). Other neurobiologic factors may be involved in individual susceptibility to dependence on particular drugs (e.g., persons with attention deficit disorder and their paradoxical relaxation with cocaine or other stimulants).

A variety of psychological perspectives applied to the level of the individual have helped us understand the psychological usefulness (and therefore, positive reinforcement) of drug effects. For example, many persons use drugs at least partly to help modulate unpleasant affects, regulate impulse control, or serve other psychological functions that healthier persons would manage without drug use. These concepts are subsumed in the "self-medication hypothesis" of drug dependence.

In addition, a wide variety of psychosocial factors influence drug use and dependence. Cultural expectations affect choice of drugs, prevalence rates, and patterns of use (e.g., binge drinking vs. chronic, moderate intake). "Culture" in this context includes that of families as well as ethnic groups, religious affiliations, subcultural identifications, nationalities, and so on. Also, drug availability, cost, and the legal and other risks associated with drug use all affect the prevalence of substance-use disorders. For example, despite the popular perception that Prohibition was a failure, and recognizing that problems existed, alcohol consumption, abuse, and dependence clearly decreased substantially in the U.S. during Prohibition.

TREATMENT

With all of this as a pathogenetic background, not surprisingly, there are a wide range of alternatives to use (singly or, more often, in combination) in the treatment of substance-use disorders. Many of these are socially based approaches that are separate from treatments offered by medical professionals (though one would hope for cooperation between the two approaches). The most prominent of these interventions is Alcoholics Anonymous (AA). Along with other self-help groups based on 12-step or similar philosophies, AA is designed to maintain abstinence and foster a sense of interpersonal (and often spiritual) connectedness in a drug-free context. Many other community, church, or other social organizations may be of use. Although varying in the degree to which they focus on the drug use itself, all provide broadly analogous support and social connectedness.

Medically based addiction programs typically offer a range of services, from inpatient detoxification or rehabilitation to day treatment programs, to less intensive varieties of outpatient contacts. Group, family, and individual psychotherapies tend to focus on:

- Breaking down the often prominent denial on the patient's part (and "enabling" behaviors by family or friends)

- Identifying the social or intrapsychic cues that signal or provoke impending relapse to drug use
- Building compensatory strategies to minimize such provocations and to manage the patient's dysphoric or otherwise unpleasant mental states without using drugs

Pharmacotherapy may play a role in the treatment of many specific drug dependencies, even beyond the role it plays in detoxification. Often medication treatment reduces craving for the abused drug (e.g., transdermal nicotine patches for cigarette smoking, naltrexone for alcoholism, methadone for opioids). Disulfiram (Antabuse) works by providing a negative reinforcer to alcohol use.

Despite some well-publicized claims to the contrary, nearly all treatment programs with documented efficacy aim for total abstinence as their goal. Although an occasional addict may be able to achieve a state of "controlled drinking" (i.e., use at nonabuse, nondependence levels), most probably cannot, and encouraging addicts en masse to aim for anything less than full abstinence usually results in colluding with their denial about the severity of their disorder.

Despite the admittedly chronic course and poor outcome for many addicts, treatments for many substance-use disorders *do* work, and large numbers of people benefit from these interventions. Aggressive treatment of comorbid psychopathology (e.g., mood or anxiety disorders) is likely to improve outcome for patients with substance dependence.

9

CHAPTER

Personality: Traits and Troubles

WHAT IS PERSONALITY?

Defining a term as complex, elusive, and allusive as "personality" is a complex, elusive, and allusive task. But in the interests of educational clarity, we won't let this stop us from trying. In a broad sense, *personality* refers to a person's enduring patterns of thinking, feeling, acting, and reacting. "Enduring" implies that personality remains fundamentally stable throughout life, and indeed, empirical research has shown that various measures of personality do remain stable from late adolescence or early adulthood into later life. Nevertheless, important changes are possible, whether facilitated by desired or undesired life events, psychotherapy, or other experiences.

Most current conceptual schemes of psychopathology consider personality as the backdrop to the development of the psychiatric disorders we have considered thus far. Often personality is an active backdrop; that is, certain personality styles or structures may put an individual at higher risk for specific psychopathology. At other times, personality may be a passive backdrop, but it colors the patient's perspectives and reactions to his or her illness and affects relationships with caregivers and providers. *The Diagnostic and Statistical Manual of Mental Disorders* (DSM-IV) continues this distinction between personality and other psychopathology: In its multiaxial diagnostic scheme, personality disorders (to be discussed below) are listed on Axis II, whereas all other psychiatric diagnoses, except for mental retardation, are listed on Axis I. This distinction can be useful, but it is arbitrary and at times difficult or impossible to make. For example, lifelong chronic depressive or anxiety symptoms, as part of a patient's everyday mental experiences, become inseparably intertwined with his or her personality. Indeed, in such cases some would argue that the patient's consequent difficulties are mislabeled as personality troubles and are really an Axis I disorder, while others would argue that the depressive or anxiety syndrome is essentially a by-product of the real problem, the Axis II difficulties. Whatever the intellectual usefulness of such debates, in clinical practice we must recognize the frequent coexistence and often the inseparability of Axis I and II disorders and treat symptomatic manifestations as best we can.

It is also crucial to recognize that acute mental states may alter what appears to be personality. For example, a person suffering with severe major depression may be needy, clingy, and dependent on others for support and reassurance but not have a dependent personality style during most (i.e., nondepressed) periods. As another example, many psychologically healthy people regress to using more rigid and dysfunctional defense mechanisms when under acute stress, such as when suffering from severe, acute medical ill-

nesses. At such times, these patients may interact with physicians in a manner that appears
typical of patients with prominent personality
disorders. The bottom line: Beware of diagnosing or labeling a patient with a personality disorder based *solely* on how they appear to you *now*.
To diagnose personality pathology, history is
needed to confirm that dysfunctional patterns
are in fact enduring, rather than artifacts of the
patient's current state.

The most prominent, and perhaps most clinically useful, perspectives for understanding personality are psychodynamic and developmentally
based. In a broad sense, personality is understood to develop during childhood from the
interplay between constitutional factors (from
genetic and prenatal influences) and life experiences. Life experiences include any obvious
stressors or traumatic events, but also includes
the nuances of the qualities of relationships with
others, beginning with parents and other primary caregivers. Of course, this interplay goes
both ways: Just as experiences shape developing
personality, so can inborn temperament shape
the responses elicited in others (e.g., it's harder
to be a consistently, calmly loving parent with an
irritable and inconsolable baby). A patient's current personality structure may be understood
using metapsychological frameworks (e.g., psychodynamics) to understand his or her common
ways of perceiving others and the world, his or
her repertoire of problem-solving strategies, predominant defense mechanisms, patterns of regu-
lating and expressing affects and impulses, and
so on.

In the course of describing these personality
characteristics (traits), labels may be useful.
Some labels (e.g., schizoid, narcissistic, or obsessive) derive directly from psychodynamic descriptions. Other schemes have been proposed to

describe personality in terms of how much or how little an individual has of each of several traits. The trick, of course, is to keep the number of traits to a manageable size and to define the traits in such fashion as to be intuitive enough to be clinically useful. Indeed, most such schemes have had greater use in research psychology than in clinical arenas. Some recent proposals have attempted to link fundamental traits with neurobiologic function (e.g., novelty seeking with dopaminergic activity), but, so far, translation to clinical practice remains elusive.

DSM-IV DEFINITIONS

An alternative (and, in practice, complementary) approach is to use categorical diagnoses. We all have personality traits, but some people have a constellation of traits that cause particular difficulty. *Personality disorders* are defined by DSM-IV as existing when personality:

- Deviates markedly from cultural expectations
- Is inflexible and pervasive across a broad range of situations
- Causes subjective distress or impairment in interpersonal relationships or other role functioning (e.g., work, school)

DSM-IV describes a number of subtypes of personality disorders based on relatively external, observable, reproducible criteria sets. The advantage of this approach is that we can diagnose personality disorders with a high degree of inter-rater reliability. Many of the resulting specific diagnoses are entities that appear to be clinically meaningful with relatively specific epidemiology, course, and treatment responses (or lack thereof).

The disadvantages of this approach are also many, including:

- Clinical richness is lacking as compared to, say, psychodynamic formulations
- Some of the entities may not be as meaningful as others.
- Many persons with clearly disordered personalities cannot be usefully categorized by a single DSM-IV diagnosis.

Given these disadvantages, it's not surprising that clinicians need to use a variety of perspectives beyond DSM-IVese to understand and work with patients with personality difficulties.

Still, it is worth becoming familiar with the basic outlines of the DSM-IV personality disorders. For convenience, they are grouped into three clusters, listed in Table 9–1. The ubiquitous NOS (not otherwise specified) is used for individuals who meet criteria for a personality dis-

Table 9–1. CLUSTERS OF PERSONALITY DISORDERS

Cluster A:
The odd or eccentric group (schizoid, schizotypal, paranoid personality disorders)

Cluster B:
The dramatic, emotional, or erratic group (borderline, narcissistic, antisocial, histrionic personality disorders)

Cluster C:
The anxious or fearful group (avoidant, dependent, obsessive-compulsive personality disorders)

order but do not meet criteria for a specific DSM-IV type. Other types of personality disorders have been described, and DSM-style criteria sets have been proposed for some, such as those appearing in the DSM-IV appendix (depressive personality disorder, passive-aggressive personality disorder). Brief descriptions of the DSM-IV disorders follow.

Cluster A (Odd or Eccentric)

Schizoid Personality Disorder

Persons with schizoid personality disorder appear eccentric because of their affective detachment and emotional coldness. They are socially isolated by choice because they do not desire or seek closeness with others. They may function well in occupational settings (typically in jobs that require little interpersonal contact or skills) but otherwise choose to lead largely solitary lives. They therefore rarely have the subjective distress or chaotic interpersonal function that leads to psychiatric contact. It should be noted that these manifestations resemble the prodromal, or negative, symptoms of schizophrenia. Thus a 20-year-old who has schizoid personality disorder may later receive a diagnosis of schizophrenia if he or she goes on to develop frank psychotic symptoms, but many persons have stable schizoid personalities throughout their lives without developing psychotic illness.

Schizotypal Personality Disorder

These persons also appear eccentric but in a more flamboyant way. They have oddities of thinking and speech, unusual ideas or beliefs, and either constricted or inappropriate affect. They also tend to be socially isolated, sometimes by preference but sometimes simply because their eccentricities drive others away, or they become fearful in social settings. By definition, however, their unusual thought processes and content do not reach frankly psychotic proportions. These persons are probably at higher risk of becoming psychotic under stress, at which point an additional Axis I diagnosis would be given to appropriately describe the psychotic syndrome.

Paranoid Personality Disorder

Persons with this disorder are, obviously, paranoid. That is, they are distrustful and suspicious of others. The main thing to recognize here is that their paranoia is *not* of delusional intensity. Again, such persons may be more likely than others to become flagrantly psychotic at times of stress, but at those times an additional diagnosis of the appropriate psychotic disorder would be made.

Cluster B (Dramatic, Emotional, or Erratic)

Borderline Personality Disorder

From the psychodynamic perspectives that led to the recognition and definition of borderline personality disorder, its fundamental underlying characteristics are:

- ⊙ A lack of a sense of self (not simply low self-esteem, but a genuine absence of a whole, integrated self image)
- ⊙ Use of primitive, maladaptive defense mechanisms such as splitting, projection, and projective identification

The term "borderline" refers to the intermediate position of such personality structure in object relations theory frameworks, between healthier "neurotic" and more impaired "psychotic" personality organizations. In the more directly observable criteria of DSM-IV, borderline personality-disordered persons manifest:

- Recurrent chaotic interpersonal relationships
- Extreme sensitivity to real or perceived abandonment
- Evidence of identity disturbance
- Chronic feelings of emptiness
- Affective instability (lifelong shifts between extremes of mood states) or frequent expressions of anger
- Self-destructive impulsivity
- Repeated or chronic suicidal ideation or directly self-injurious actions
- Transient psychotic symptoms (including paranoid delusions or hallucinations) during periods of stress

Persons at the healthier end of the borderline personality disorder spectrum may maintain jobs and long-term relationships with others, albeit with considerable subjective distress and some degree of interpersonal turmoil underneath their more functional surface. Patients with more severe forms, however, are often high users of psychiatric (and medical) services and, unsurprisingly, form difficult, chaotic relationships with their caregivers. The considerable affect often evoked in caregivers must be monitored carefully if appropriate, professional, effective treatments are to be provided.

Narcissistic Personality Disorder

The most prominent characteristics of persons with this disorder are

- Evidence of grandiosity of thoughts or behavior

- Need for recognition of their self-perceived specialness
- Lack of empathy for others

Many persons with this disorder also meet criteria for other personality disorders. Looking from a psychodynamic perspective, one can see the hollow core underneath the grandiose bluster of pathological narcissism. In other words, many (perhaps most or all) persons with narcissistic personality have borderline personality–type organization, with a concomitant lack of sense of self and propensity for primitive, maladaptive defenses. Unlike "pure" borderline personalities, however, narcissistic persons cover up their borderline core with a shell of grandiosity. This cover has its advantages: Narcissistic personalities are much less prone to affective instability, poor impulse control, or suicidal tendencies than are pure borderline personalities. But because the grandiose shell is thin and hollow, it requires constant reinforcement to keep it intact, and interpersonal relationships come to be viewed solely in terms of how much they help maintain the grandiose image by admiration, recognition of specialness, and so on.

Antisocial Personality Disorder

The cardinal feature of this disorder is pervasive disregard for and violation of the rights of others. Manifestations include chronic lying or other deceitfulness, lawbreaking, and irresponsibility. Impulsivity, irritability, or aggressiveness, and novelty-seeking actions (with disregard for safety of self or others) may be present. Lack of remorse, often accompanied by externalizing blame, is characteristic. By definition, persons with this disorder must show evidence of conduct disorder before age 15 years, with manifestations essentially being the childhood equivalents of adult antisocial behaviors. Antisocial personalities, commonly termed *sociopaths* or *psychopaths* in the lay media, can appear charismatically charming or ingratiating if doing so serves their immediate needs. They also often appear to be wholly without anxiety or worries of any sort. Beneath their surface smoothness and confidence, though, is an emptiness that is not often or easily apparent, since relationships with others tend to be brief and superficial. Antisocial personality disorder is more common in men, is quite prevalent in prison populations, and is often comorbid with substance-use disorders. Patients are unlikely to benefit from treatment by traditional psychiatric settings and methods, since by definition their relationships with others are wholly built around exploitation to gratify their immediate needs.

Histrionic Personality Disorder

The main characteristics of this disorder are excessive emotionality (theatrical) and attention seeking. Despite striking displays of affect, there is often a superficial quality to emotional life and relationships. Persons with this disorder may be quite suggestible and impulsive in their beliefs and actions. Flirtatious or otherwise sexually provocative styles are often used to help draw attention to themselves. At the healthier end of the spectrum, patients with histrionic personality disorder retain the capacity for relatively unambivalent intimacy, which allows them to make successful use of psychodynamic psychotherapy. At the more severe end of the spectrum, the histrionic style may in fact be underlined by more fundamental troubles with sense of self (i.e., borderline personality organization), with attendant greater difficulties in interpersonal relationships, including psychotherapies.

Cluster C (Anxious or Fearful)

Avoidant Personality Disorder

The core feature of this disorder is a pattern of social inhibition, related to feelings of inadequacy and fears of being criticized, shamed, or rejected. There is considerable overlap between this disorder and generalized social phobia. Often both diagnoses apply, and they may in fact be the same or similar conditions. (Translation: More research might lead to one of them being eliminated from future DSMs.) For now, though, social phobia is defined a bit more narrowly (i.e., anxiety while actually facing social situations), whereas avoidant personality disorder is defined in terms of broader preoccupations with self-image as related to others.

Dependent Personality Disorder

Persons with dependent personality disorder have an excessive need to be taken care of, which leads to submissive and clinging behavior and fears of being left alone. Dependent behaviors are common in many other personality disorders and in other disorders such as major depression. In dependent personality disorder, however, the dependency features are pervasive and enduring (e.g., present not only when patient is depressed), and the more specific neediness of other personality disorders (e.g., narcissists requiring admiration) is lacking.

Obsessive-Compulsive Personality Disorder

Persons with this disorder demonstrate a preoccupation with details, orderliness, and perfectionism as a means to maintaining control over mental activity and interpersonal events. (Note that here the term "obsessiveness" retains its familiar meaning from lay usage, different from the obsessions of obsessive-compulsive disorder.) Of course, some degree of obsessiveness is useful to completing tasks and achieving goals. In obsessive-compulsive personality disorder, however, the obsessiveness is at the expense of flexibility, openness, and efficiency. The major point of activities may be lost, tasks may not be completed, and relationships beyond those needed for work and productivity are often impaired.

Passive-Aggressive Personality Disorder

This disorder is *not* an official DSM-IV diagnosis. It is listed in the appendix as a criteria set for further study. Whatever remains to be done to validate specific criteria for a particular personality disorder, however, the *concept* of passive-aggressive style is worth mentioning because it is a common and troublesome dynamic seen in persons with other personality disorders (and in some without). It is characterized by a pervasive pattern of negativistic attitudes and passive resistance to demands for adequate performance. Typically there is a combination of passively failing to complete tasks (e.g., by "forgetting," or indefinite procrastination), along with a tendency to blame others and deny responsibility for lack of accomplishments. In other words, these persons actively control their lives and environment through inaction.

TREATMENT

Personality disorders are by definition chronic. Also, by the nature of most of them, patients tend to see the problems as others' fault and have difficulty accepting responsibility for their own recurrent pattern of action. The less psychologically minded may not even see a recurrent pattern, let alone understand their role in perpetuating it. For all these reasons, treatment of personality disorders has a rather hopeless reputation in many quarters. And indeed, empirical research has shown that personality remains remarkably stable throughout adulthood.

Still, being realistic does not mean being hopeless. Most persons with personality disorders who present in psychiatric clinical settings are suffering from a comorbid Axis I disorder; that is, their internal mental state has changed, often related to a change in external circumstances or stressors. Common comorbidities include mood, anxiety, and substance-use disorders, although sometimes the stress-related clinical exacerbation is best captured by a diagnosis of "merely" an adjustment disorder. Aggressive treatment of comorbid Axis I conditions is essential and helpful. Also (and of primary importance in adjustment disorders), crisis-oriented psychotherapy, including supportive and cognitive-behavioral techniques, can help patients regain their psychological homeostasis by using their healthier defenses and minimizing their less healthy or more destructive patterns.

Longer-term psychotherapy is indicated for patients whose disorders are severe enough to lead to behavioral sequelae that bring them into frequent contact with acute mental health services (e.g., recurrent suicide attempts). Patients with less severe disorders may seek psychotherapy to ameliorate what they perceive as dysfunctional patterns of behavior—a recognition that, by itself, is a good prognostic sign. It is beyond the scope of this section, or of this book, to detail the techniques of the psychotherapy itself, which in fact must vary considerably along the supportive-expressive continuum in relation to the specific personality disorder, developmental phase, assessments of the integrity of self, and so on. Given the enormous number of difficult-to-quantify variables, empirical research on long-term outcome of psychotherapy with personality disorders is rather sparse. Long-standing clinical experience supports its overall usefulness, but parameters for optimal efficacy or cost effectiveness are not known.

Pharmacotherapy has a place in some patients, particularly at times of crisis. Neuroleptics may be used to target transient psychotic or near-psychotic symptoms in patients with schizotypal, paranoid, or borderline personality disorders. Neuroleptics may also have a role in the short-term management of severe impulse or affect "dyscontrol" in severe cluster B disorders. Thymoleptics such as lithium and carbamazepine may be helpful in the longer run for affective instability or impulsivity in any personality disorder. Antidepressants and anxiolytics also have their uses, but these should be guided mostly by Axis I comorbidities.

10
CHAPTER

Somatoform Disorders and Other Psychopathological Categories

Patients frequently present to physicians of all specialties with physical symptoms that cannot be explained in kind or degree by identifiable physical pathology. Any of a number of psychiatric disorders may or may not help explain the patient's presentation. The clinical and differential diagnostic approach to such situations will be discussed in Chapter 19. Here, let's briefly review the relevant *Diagnostic and Statistical Manual of Mental Disorders* (DSM-IV) categories that we have not yet covered.

PSYCHOLOGICAL FACTORS AFFECTING MEDICAL CONDITION

This is not a mental disorder per se, but is important enough to be listed in DSM-IV anyway. The basic point here is that known, diagnosable physical disorders may be affected by emotional or psychological processes in various ways, as shown by these examples:

- Anxiety contributing to symptoms of a medical illness (e.g., the gastrointestinal hypermotility of irritable bowel syndrome)
- Stress-induced worsening of primary medical conditions (e.g., angina, diabetic hyperglycemia, asthmatic bronchospasm)
- Health-related behaviors affecting medical course (e.g., lifestyle activities that are risks for the onset or worsening of specific medical disorders)

MALINGERING

Malingering also is not a mental disorder, but it certainly is a troublesome behavior and, as such, is listed in DSM-IV. In malingering, the patient consciously and intentionally produces false or grossly exaggerated physical or psychological symptoms—in other words, lies. The patient does so with some specific external goal in mind, which may be obtaining money (e.g., lawsuits or workers compensation), avoiding an undesired duty (job, prison term), or obtaining drugs. Malingering should be suspected if strong external incentives favor symptom production, if the symptoms are difficult to reconcile with objective findings, if compliance with diagnostic or therapeutic recommendations is poor, and if the patient has other evidence for antisocial personality disorder. However, unless the patient's lie is directly exposed, it can sometimes be difficult to diagnose malingering with certainty.

FACTITIOUS DISORDERS

Factitious disorders are officially classified as mental disorders in DSM-IV. The patient intentionally feigns or produces physical or psychological symptoms or signs, with the sole motivation of assuming the sick role. (That is, external motivations such as found in malingering are absent.) When physical symptoms are produced, this disorder is more commonly known as *Munchausen's syndrome*. Examples of sign production include placing a drop of blood in one's urine, leading to workup for hematuria; self-injecting foreign materials to produce low-grade fevers, or insulin to produce hypoglycemia; and surreptitiously ingesting anticoagulants to produce bleeding. As a result of these presentations, patients with Munchausen's syndrome may undergo numerous invasive diagnostic or therapeutic procedures. Munchausen's syndrome is more common in women. Patients often have some history of employment in the health professions or other connection with them, which may permit access to needed equipment such as syringes and also provides the knowledge base needed to produce symptoms that are sufficiently alarming to warrant workup. Some adult patients produce symptoms in their children and seek pediatric attention, a condition known as *Munchausen's by proxy*.

The obvious question this clinical picture raises is, why would anyone do all this merely to assume the sick role? Unfortunately, such patients tend to resist psychiatric intervention or even contact. Indeed, when confronted with their behavior, they tend to react indignantly and resist further evaluation. Also, although they are consciously aware of what they are doing to produce symptoms, they typically are not aware of their motivation. Thus, speculation about etiology is just that—speculation—although complex unconscious factors are almost certainly involved. Prominent psychodynamics probably include the desire to be taken care of and form close relationships with health care professionals, or the expression of hostility toward health care professionals (by "tricking" them) and themselves (by subjecting themselves to uncomfortable or dangerous procedures).

Optimal treatment of factitious disorder probably should involve both setting limits on the symptom-producing behavior (via confrontation or behavioral therapies), and psychodynamic psychotherapy to address the underlying character issues that led to the need for seeking care or expressing rage in such dysfunctional fashion. Treatment tends to be difficult, however, even for the few patients who allow any psychiatric contact. An additional strategy may include alerting nearby hospitals and emergency rooms to the patient's presentation, with the goal of raising the level of suspicion and reducing unnecessary tests, procedures, or surgeries.

SOMATOFORM DISORDERS

Several somatoform disorders are listed in DSM-IV. It is most important to understand their overall commonality. The distinctions among most of them are substantially historical or arbitrary, so although descriptions of the specific diagnoses are provided below, these details are less crucial for most clinicians than the general principles.

In general, patients with somatoform disorders have distressing physical symptoms that are either unrelated to or grossly in excess of what would be expected from identifiable medical conditions. The symptoms are *not*—repeat, *not*—consciously feigned or produced; these patients are not malingering, nor do they have a factitious disorder. Psychological factors are generally presumed to be contributory to the physical symptoms in somatoform disorders, although DSM-IV explicitly asks only for clinician judgment that this is so only for conversion and pain disorders, probably because the evidence for such judgments is rather hard to define operationally.

The basic types of somatoform disorders are:

- *Somatization disorder,* also known as *Briquet's syndrome.* Patients with this disorder have numerous somatoform symptoms from multiple organ systems over many years. Therefore, chronicity is inherently built into the diagnosis. This disorder is more prevalent in women, and comorbidity with personality disorders and other Axis I disorders (e.g., substance use, anxiety disorders) is common.
- *Pain disorder,* which is essentially a mono-symptomatic somatoform condition, with the predominant symptom being pain (surprising, no?).
- *Conversion disorder,* another (usually) mono-symptomatic somatoform condition. The symptom is an alteration in voluntary motor or sensory function, typically suggestive of neurological disease. Examples include conversion blindness, paralysis, or seizures ("pseudoseizures").
- *Undifferentiated somatoform disorder,* perhaps the most grab-bag category among the somatoform disorders. This disorder includes patients with somatoform symptoms that are (1) *not* predominantly pain or mo-

tor/sensory, and (2) not sufficient in number
or duration to meet criteria for full-fledged
somatization disorder. Thus, patients in this
category range from those with one transient symptom to those with multiple symptoms just shy of Briquet's-level presentation.
DSM-IV does require that the symptom(s)
last at least 6 months; shorter-term symptoms fall under the even more heterogeneous term *Somatoform Disorder Not Otherwise Specified.*

- *Hypochondriasis,* which, unlike the above
  somatoform disorders, is not defined by
  symptom presentation. Hypochondriasis is
  defined as you would expect from its lay
  connotation: undue worry about having a
  serious disease, based on misinterpretation
  of normal or abnormal bodily symptoms or
  functions. By definition, the worry cannot be
  of delusional proportions, but it typically
  leads to frequent contact with medical or
  other health care professionals, whose reassurances fail to assuage the patient.
- *Body dysmorphic disorder,* in which patients
  become preoccupied with imagined or
  greatly exaggerated defects in their physical
  appearance. The preoccupation may involve
  any body part. Examples include unrealistic
  worry about thinning hair, a large or
  crooked nose, or genital size or appearance.
  Patients may seek physical remedies from
  dermatologists, plastic surgeons, or other
  specialists for the perceived defects. Body
  dysmorphic disorder may be qualitatively
  distinct from the other somatoform disorders in that it may be pathogenically related
  to obsessive-compulsive disorder, as suggested by recent evidence of partial improvement with serotonin reuptake inhibitors.

An approach to the differential diagnosis of

patients with unexplained physical symptoms, including the assessment and management of somatoform disorders, is thoughtfully provided in Chapter 19.

OTHER PSYCHOPATHOLOGIC CATEGORIES

The following is a very brief tour through the remaining categories in DSM-IV. The descriptions are quite limited and therefore cannot do justice to these complex entities, which have been lumped together here under "other" because mastery of these areas is less important for most trainees rotating on psychiatry services for the first time, as compared with the disorders already considered. Sleep disorders and developmental and child psychiatry disorders are discussed in Chapter 19.

Eating Disorders

Eating disorders are, obviously, defined by abnormalities in eating behavior. There are two main types:

- *Anorexia nervosa:* These patients fail to maintain a minimally normal weight for their age and height, through some combination of limiting caloric intake, exercising to burn off calories, or purging activities (self-induced vomiting; misuse of laxatives, enemas, or diuretics). They have a distorted sense of their own body weight, shape, or image and hence fear gaining weight even when they are dangerously underweight. Postmenarcheal girls also have amenorrhea.

- *Bulimia nervosa:* These patients do maintain adequate weight but have recurrent episodes of binge eating, defined as discrete periods of large food intake along with a sense of lack of control of the intake. They also exhibit behaviors intended to compensate for the binges and prevent weight gain, such as purging, fasting, or excessive exercise. Persons with this disorder also have distorted self-images of their bodies, or excessively tie their overall self-image to their perception of their body shape or size.

Dissociative Disorders

Dissociative disorders are defined by the presence of dissociative symptoms—that is, disruptions in otherwise normal-functioning consciousness, memory, identity, or environmental perception. Note that dissociative symptoms may occur as part of other disorders, such as post-traumatic and acute stress disorders. The primary dissociative disorders include:

- *Dissociative amnesia,* one or more episodes of memory loss (often of stressful or traumatic events) that cannot be explained by a physical or another mental disorder.
- *Dissociative fugue,* in which patients suddenly and unexpectedly travel away from their usual environments and either assume a new identity or are confused about their past experiences and identity.
- *Dissociative identity disorder,* formerly and still popularly known as *multiple personality disorder.* This disorder is characterized by shifts among two or more distinct identities or personality states, each of which has its own enduring patterns of thinking, feeling,

and acting. (Think of popular media examples such as *Sybil* or *The Three Faces of Eve*.)

There's considerable debate regarding the prevalence or even the existence of true dissociative identity disorder. Clearly, some patients display different "alters" (identities), sometimes in dramatic fashion, but whether these patients truly have psychopathology distinguishable from other mental disorders (such as borderline personality disorder), and how much the creation of alters depends on psychotherapist expectations, is quite controversial.

- *Depersonalization disorder,* episodes of feeling physically and mentally detached from one's own mind and body. Again, depersonalization is a symptom that may also be seen in other mental disorders such as acute stress or panic disorder.
- *Dissociative disorder NOS,* a term used for even less well-defined, or more unusual, cases of dissociation, such as what used to be called "psychogenic unresponsiveness."

Paraphilias

Paraphilias are characterized by recurrent, intense, and distressing or impairing sexual fantasies, urges, or behaviors. They typically involve nonhuman or nonconsenting objects, or the humiliation of oneself or one's partner. Specific types include:

- *Exhibitionism*—exposing one's genitals to strangers
- *Fetishism*—arousal from inanimate objects such as undergarments
- *Frotteurism*—touching or rubbing against nonconsenting persons

- *Pedophilia*—sexually arousing fantasies, urges, or actions involving prepubescent children
- *Sexual masochism*—arousal related to being beaten, humiliated, or otherwise suffering
- *Sexual sadism*—arousal related to similar suffering inflicted on others
- *Transvestic fetishism*—arousal involving cross-dressing
- *Voyeurism*—arousal involving watching naked, disrobing, or sexually active, unsuspecting other persons

Sexual Dysfunctions

Sexual dysfunctions are defined as impairments in sexual desire or in the psychophysiology of the sexual response cycle. They may be lifelong or of more recent onset and may be generalized or limited to specific situations. Sexual dysfunctions may be caused by known physiological factors (e.g., secondary sexual dysfunctions due to general medical conditions or substance-induced syndromes), psychological factors, or both. The primary (largely psychological) dysfunctions may be organized as follows, based partly on the phase of the sexual response cycle affected:

- *Sexual desire disorders*—hypoactive sexual desire, sexual aversion disorder
- *Disorders of sexual arousal*—male erectile or female arousal disorders
- *Orgasmic disorders*—trouble attaining orgasm (female or male orgasmic disorders) and premature ejaculation
- *Sexual pain disorders*—dyspareunia and vaginismus (considered mental disorders only if not due to medical illnesses)

Gender Identity Disorder

Gender identity disorder is characterized by pervasive cross-gender identification and discomfort with one's actual gender. This means not merely cross-dressing but a strong desire to behave in stereotypic cross-gender manners or to be the other gender. Some persons with this disorder, particularly those with onset in childhood, seek sex-reassignment surgery.

Impulse Control Disorders

Impulse-control disorders are defined by the failure to resist an impulse, drive, or temptation to perform an act that is harmful to self or others. For many, the act is preceded by a growing sense of tension or arousal and is followed by pleasure or relief. There may or may not be guilt or regrets. These diagnoses are used only if the poor impulse control is not explained by another mental disorder (e.g., fire setting as part of a psychotic disorder). Specific categories include the following:

- *Kleptomania*—recurrent senseless stealing of objects
- *Pyromania*—fire setting
- *Pathological gambling*—broadly analogous in its clinical features to an addiction, although physiological dependence is obviously lacking
- *Trichotillomania*—pulling of one's own hair, which may have clinical or neurobiologic overlap with obsessive-compulsive disorder
- *Intermittent explosive disorder*—discrete episodes of aggressivity; however, there is considerable controversy as to whether or not this genuinely exists as a discrete disorder separate from other psychopathology

Adjustment Disorders

Adjustment disorders are manifested by clinically significant emotional or behavioral symptoms that occur in direct response to specific stressful events. The symptoms must resolve within 6 months after the resolution of the stressor. This diagnosis is not given if the symptoms meet criteria for another Axis I condition, since stressful events often precipitate other mental disorders. Thus, someone who develops six depressive symptoms for a 4-week period after being fired would be diagnosed with major depression, *not* with an adjustment disorder. Various specifiers are given to describe the nature of the symptoms, such as adjustment disorder with depressed mood, with anxiety, with mixed anxiety and depressed mood, with disturbance of conduct, with mixed disturbance of emotions and conduct, and the ubiquitous "unspecified."

3
PART

The Psychiatric Workup

This section describes the kinds of data you will need to obtain as you evaluate psychiatric patients and offers guidelines on how to organize these data. You'll also need to explicate what you think about your patients' presentations and what you plan to do to intervene. Guidelines are provided here for these things as well.

11
CHAPTER

The History and Physical Examination

The good news is that the psychiatric workup is similar in broad outline, and in many details, to the general medical workup you've been doing all along. The bad news—well, there really is no bad news. But there are important points of refinement that, although applicable to other settings, will be especially highlighted in psychiatry. And you will have to become accustomed to, and skilled at, gathering and organizing psychological and psychosocial data with the degree of detail and rigor that you are used to employing with physical symptoms, laboratory values, and other supposedly objective data. ("Supposedly" because seemingly hard data such as liver span by percussion or sphygmomanometer-obtained blood pressures can vary considerably; indeed, as mentioned earlier, psychiatric syndromes can be ascertained with the same degree of reliability as most general medical data.)

An outline of a psychiatric workup is provided in Table 11–1. What follows in this and the next two chapters is a blow-by-blow description of the kinds of things to consider as you complete each section.

Table 11–1. PSYCHIATRIC WORKUP

Identifying Data: Age, race, gender, marital status, referred by whom for what?

Chief Complaint: Patient's perception of the main problem

History of Present Illness: Presenting symptoms organized syndromically if possible, and their chronology/context

Medications: List all

Past Psychiatric History: Substance-use history; prior psychiatric syndromes, treatments (including psychotropic medication history)

Past Medical and Surgical History: The usual

Family History: Psychiatric and medical family history; genogram; family relationship patterns

Developmental/Social History: Role performances throughout life course; current living and social circumstances

Review of Systems: The basic medical ROS, plus any relevant psychiatric ROS not already covered

Physical Examination: The usual, but pay careful attention to the neurological exam

Mental Status Examination: A significant part of what you're here to learn. Components include

General appearance and behavior
Quality of relationship to interviewer
Psychomotor activity
Speech
Mood and affect
Thought content
Thought process
Perceptual disturbances
Cognitive functions
  Level of consciousness
  Orientation
  Attention
  Memory
  Language
  Fund of knowledge
  Visuospatial skills
  Calculations
  Frontal executive functions
  Abstraction
Judgment and insight

Table 11–1. *Continued*

Laboratory Values: All current (and any recent and relevant) blood work, neuroimaging studies, etc.
Diagnostic Impressions: The Five Axes of *DSM-IV*
Formulation: How do you understand both the nature and the potential etiology of the patient's presenting problems?
Problem List and Plan: All relevant psychiatric and medical problems, and all relevant biological, psychological, and social interventions

IDENTIFYING DATA

As with the usual medical workup, the identifying data should be a brief sentence or two that tells who the patient is (in a nonprofound, demographic sense) and how and why the patient has presented for evaluation or treatment. For "how," it is often useful to describe the method of referral, particularly whether the patient was self-referred or sent by a general medical provider or another mental health professional. For inpatient workups, a statement of the patient's admission status (e.g., voluntary, involuntary) will help convey a sense of the referral process and the patient's response to this process. As to the "why," be brief but descriptive of *your* sense of the most important or prominent part of the patient's presentation.

CHIEF COMPLAINT

Here's the patient's chance to get in a few words as to what *he or she* sees as most important or prominent. Use direct quotes or paraphrases whenever possible. Often in psychiatry, comparison between the identifying data and the chief complaint is illuminating. For example, ID–This is a 26-year-old single white male admitted from the emergency department on an involuntary status with paranoid psychosis. CC—"There's nothing wrong with me—you should be locking up my neighbors after what they did to me!"

HISTORY OF PRESENT ILLNESS

In principle, this section is straightforward. After all, all you have to do is describe what the patient is presenting with, right? In practice, of course, probably more thought, care, and effort will go into this section than anything else in the workup (except perhaps for the formulation).

Let's start with sources of information. You'll have to learn what you can from the patient, which, depending on the setting and the patient's psychiatric acuity, will vary from the whole story to pieces of the story (with varying degrees of accuracy), to none of it (in the cases of mute, uncooperative, or incoherent patients, which odds are you'll encounter at some point during the rotation). There may be other medical or psychiatric records to review that will shed light on the history of present illness (HPI) as well as be directly relevant to past history (see below). In most acute settings, be it inpatient psychiatry, medical floor consultations, or the emergency department, you will want or need to supplement the history by speaking with other informants. These informants may include the referring or consultation-requesting caregivers, or family, friends, or others who know the patient well (or at least better than you do). Needless to say, even in these days of cellular telephones and fax machines, it may take time to gather the full database; it is not uncommon for the whole process to take several days after a complex inpatient admission. At some point you're going to have to bite the bullet and write up what data you have, knowing that it will be supplemented or supplanted by what you will eventually learn. Accept these limitations calmly and humbly—they go with the territory—and make clear in the beginning of your workup what your data sources are and what your best estimate is of the data's reliability and completeness. (You can also note in your plan section what you intend to do to complete the database.)

The next tough issue is to decide when the HPI begins. This is easy for patients with new, recent-onset illness (e.g., "Mr. Jones was in his usual state of excellent health until 3 weeks ago, when he began to develop the following symptoms. . ."). It's not so easy for patients with prior episodes, symptoms, or treatment encounters. However, the issue is exactly analogous to what you've encountered in medical settings. For example, if Ms. Robinson is being admitted to your care in the intensive care unit with an acute myocardial infarction, does the HPI begin with the severe pain and dyspnea she developed 4 hours ago? Does it begin with the escalating angina symptoms she's had over the past 2 weeks? Or does it begin with her coronary artery bypass grafting last year? Well, the same questions arise in psychiatry: Does the HPI begin with Mr. Felschmidt's escalating psychotic symptoms and suicidal focus over the 6 hours before coming to the emergency department? Does it begin with his binge use of cocaine over the past 6 days? Or does it begin with his admission for newly diagnosed schizophrenia last year? The bottom line is that there is no one right way to do your HPI. In theory, you can start anywhere that logically connects to the current presentation. In practice, though, you're more likely to be able to tightly organize and present your data if you limit the HPI as much as is clinically sensible. For Mr.

Felschmidt, it is probably prudent to include his binge cocaine use in the HPI because it probably contributed to the exacerbation of his psychotic symptoms (as you'll argue later in your formulation). But you can state in the HPI that he has a past history of schizophrenia and leave it at that for now, since the details of this history fall naturally under "past psychiatric history."

Once you've decided on a temporal starting point, you still need an organizing principle for your HPI. The most common organizer used by neophytes is chronology. That is, one reports what happened first, then next, and next, and so on, up to the events directly leading to presentation. Of course, some filtering of data is required since some of what happens next may fit better under social history, or may not be relevant to the clinical context at all. The advantage of this approach is its simplicity. You don't need to have an overarching conception of the patient's illness to present the HPI, you just "tell it like it was." This is also the chronological approach's great disadvantage. To develop a conception of the patient's illness after examining such an HPI, the reader must pull data together from disparate parts of the chronology.

The chronological approach *can* be used successfully and is probably the only way to go when you have no idea how to pull the history together in a meaningful way. Most of the best and tightest HPIs take a different tack, however, one that we'll call the *syndromic approach*. An analogy may help illustrate the basic idea here. A strong workup should be argued like a legal brief. The strands of the history and physical—in the HPI's case, pertinent positives and negatives—should be filtered and organized so as to lead inexorably to the closing "argument," the formulation and differential diagnosis. By the time you get to your formulation, the links to the preceding database should be so clear that the formulation leaps out as obviously correct and fully supported. You won't actually conclude with "I rest my case," but, in fact, a well organized workup *does* say this in effect.

So how does one translate all this metaphorical rhetoric into action? Remember that the key to psychiatric differential diagnosis involves clustering symptoms into recognizable syndromes as much as possible. Begin the HPI with a terse description of the patient's presenting symptoms, clustered together as much as possible. (For example, "Ms. Xanadu developed depressive symptoms including persistently depressed mood with daily crying spells, feelings of worthlessness, early morning awakening by 2 hours, and weight loss of 17 pounds. . . . She also noted increasing 'nervousness,' which was present continuously but with some variation in degree. Along with this anxiety, she had dry mouth, tremulousness, and nausea. . . .") As part of your symptom descriptions, you will want to include relevant "dimensions" of the symptoms, including severity, time course, aggravating or alleviating factors, and other associated symptoms, just as you would for a physical symptom. Also, use terse examples to help flesh out your descriptions: After mentioning that a patient had persecutory delusions, convey the content of these delusions (e.g., "He felt that his neighbors had tried to poison his food").

You also will want to describe the context within which the patient experiences symptoms. Context might include the immediate setting (e.g., anxiety first noticed immediately after a disruptive argument with spouse) as well as the more general stressors or significant events that have taken place during the time of the presenting symptoms (e.g., 5 or 6 weeks of escalating depressive symptoms, during which time the patient has faced several difficult-to-meet deadlines at work and also learned of the death of a cousin). It is important not to make premature attributions of *causality* in relation to stressors. Don't say in the HPI, "The patient became depressed because of pressures at work." Save such causal speculation for the formulation. On the other hand, it *is* helpful to include patient attributions, such as "The patient felt that these worsening depressive symptoms were due to the stress at work."

The HPI is also a place to include "pertinent negatives." If the patient presents with severe depression, and you've already described seven or eight depressive symptoms that are present, it is useful to mention the depressive symptoms that are absent (e.g., no suicidal thinking or diurnal variation). If the patient has delusions, mention explicitly whether or not they have other psychotic symptoms (i.e., hallucinations, gross thought process disruption). As in any medical workup, the differential diagnosis drives whether or not a "negative" is truly pertinent. Thus, your selection of pertinent negatives will buttress your differential diagnostic formulation later on, in keeping with the legal brief model discussed above.

Having detailed the patient's symptoms, it is now helpful to use a chronological approach to describe what the patient tried to do for his or her symptoms. This might include a description of recent treatments given, such as, "He saw his primary care physician, who prescribed fluoxetine 20 mg po qd, but the patient self-discontinued this after 1 week because of increased nausea and lack of improvement in his depressive symptoms." This description should also clearly explicate how the patient came to present to you today: For example, "He made an appointment with my psychiatry preceptor's office on the recommendation of his primary care physician due to continued worsening anxiety," or, "Her daughter called the police after being threatened with a knife by the patient, and the police arrested the patient under state mental hygiene law and brought her to the emergency department."

MEDICATIONS

A full list of all medications, with dosage schedules if known, is essential. Indicate if compliance for certain drugs, or for all of them, is questionable or lacking. Also describe any recent changes in regimen—"Haloperidol 5 mg po qhs begun yesterday in the emergency room; perphenazine 8 mg po qhs was previously prescribed." Don't forget to inquire about all psychotropic and other medications. Also, ask specifically about over-the-counter drugs, vitamins, and topical agents (skin creams, eye drops, etc.).

PAST PSYCHIATRIC HISTORY

After listing medications, describe here the patient's substance-use history (unless you've already placed this information in the HPI because of its relevance to the presenting problem). In any case, describe what substances are used, doses or amounts, and chronology (including frequency and pattern of use), and review pertinent positives and negatives regarding abuse and dependence—for instance, has he or she had alcoholic blackouts, withdrawal symptoms, or attempts to cut down or quit usage? Also describe any formal outpatient or inpatient substance-use treatments.

N.B.: You've probably been taught elsewhere to put substance use under "Social History," but doing so demeans the direct relevance of substance use to physical and mental disorders. You *may* find it helpful to describe under Social History the social circumstances in which the patient uses drugs, such as drinking routinely after work with coworkers or only on weekends with a spouse.

You can then proceed to detail any other past psychiatric history. You'll need to ask the patient about this in several ways to get a complete picture. Has he or she ever seen a psychiatrist or other mental health professional? ("Counselor" and "therapist" are words that may trigger patient recall.) Has the patient ever been counseled by a primary physician for emotional troubles? Been given a "nerve pill" or a "sleeping pill" by any doctor? Been hospitalized for emotional or psychiatric reasons? Tried to harm or kill himself or herself in the past? (It's surprising how many people will tell you "yes" to this, after denying all prior queries about emotional troubles or treatments.) A review of office or hospital records can be essential in further clarifying these issues. Also, any "yes" answers should lead to a series of questions designed to elicit specifics, including:

- What diagnoses were given?
- What specific symptoms were present?
- What treatments were used? (Including details of medication trials—doses, duration, adverse effects)
- Response to treatments and the subsequent course (did they return to baseline?)

In addition to formal history of psychiatric treatments, it is essential to ask about relevant past syndromes that may have been untreated and long since forgotten by the patient. For example, if Ms. Fratelli, a 29-year-old single white woman, presents with delusional depression, it is crucial to know if she has previously suffered from depressive or manic episodes. If she denies formal contacts in the past, it is necessary to specifically ask her and any other knowledgeable informants questions such as: "Was there ever a time in your life when you felt sad or blue much of the time for at least a couple of weeks on end? What about a period when you just felt less interested in things?" (Follow up any "yes" responses with further queries about particular depressive symptoms and chronology.) Also ask, "Have you ever had distinct periods in your life when your mood was unusually happy, giddy, or 'on top of the world'?" (Follow up with queries about other manic symptoms as indicated.)

PAST MEDICAL AND SURGICAL HISTORY

You've spent the rest of your training learning how to do this section, so we won't dwell on the details. But please remember not to skimp on this section just because it's a "psych patient." Medical illnesses are *highly* comorbid with psychiatric disorders and are often directly relevant (physiologically or otherwise) to the psychiatric presentation.

FAMILY HISTORY

In principle, this section should be no different from what you've done in other settings. In practice, though, along with the usual genogram showing who's who and has what physical disorders, be sure to ask specifically about family histories of psychiatric disorders. Just as for past psychiatric history, you may have to do some creative (i.e., clear and specific) questioning not only about formal contacts with the mental health care system, but about untreated syndromes, hospitalizations (which in the "old days" might have meant institutionalization), suicide attempts or completions, and alcohol or other substance-use troubles. If you do elicit a family history, ideally you'd like to know details of symptoms, diagnoses, and treatments (including specific medications), although often family members don't know the details about, say, why Uncle Lou was "put away," thanks in part to the stigma attached to mental illness.

Also, this is a good place in your workup to consider the relationships among family members, although in an initial workup of acute patients you may have little information in this regard at first. Still, you will want to make note of relevant aspects of the family's cultural, socioeconomic, or religious background, prominent or enduring patterns of (mis)communication, and areas of particular alliance or discord among family members, especially between the patient and others.

DEVELOPMENTAL/SOCIAL HISTORY

Developmental history is of fundamental importance to a full psychodynamic understanding of the patient and may also yield helpful clues as to the etiology or clinical phenomenology of the current condition. For these reasons, it is important that you develop expertise in obtaining and presenting these data, although under certain circumstances obtaining a full developmental history may be unnecessary (e.g., an emergency room visit) or impossible (e.g., a mute or assaultive patient). Previous psychiatric or medical records may help in these, and indeed, in all circumstances.

In any case, a useful perspective to help organize your developmental history is the concept of *role performance*. We each fulfill several roles simultaneously at each stage of our lives. To pick a random example, one might be a parent, spouse, son, teacher, clinician, researcher, and so on, at the same time. Role performance depends on many factors, including intelligence, innate aptitudes, learned skills, personality characteristics, and acute or chronic psychiatric or medical disorders. Some people perform some of these roles more successfully than others. It is therefore helpful to tease apart function in different domains (e.g., social, occupational, academic, etc.).

A full developmental history starts with noting if there were any complications in utero; that is, were there any troubles during the pregnancy or delivery of the patient? Next, successful development may be evidenced by the patient's achieving motor, cognitive, and social milestones of early childhood (those you learned from studying human development and pediatrics). As a coarse screen in working with an adult, ask if the patient walked, talked, and in general did the things kids do on schedule, or were there any delays? Proceeding to the patient's school years, ask about academic role performance:

- Did the patient complete grades as scheduled?
- Did he or she require special or remedial education?
- What specific grades did he or she get?

Also ask about social roles:

- What kind of network of friends did the patient have in school?
- How did he or she relate to parents, siblings, or others in the household?

These same topics apply as you ask about adolescence, with the addition of questions about romantic and sexual relationships:

- Ask about dating or other similar acts.
- Specifically, take a sexual history.

Moving on to early adulthood, domains of concern include social and occupational:

- Spouse or other love/sexual relationships
- Friends
- Community, religious, sports, or hobbies-related organizations
- Other avocational group affiliations
- A careful job history, noting any patterns of difficulty with maintaining employment and trying to specify what led to any troubles (i.e., interpersonal conflict, inability to do the work effectively, etc.).

Continue these tacks as you move through adulthood, inquiring specifically about how the patient performed developmental tasks and reacted to expected or unexpected stressful events over the years (e.g., raising children, illnesses, financial or other losses, children leaving the household, job promotions or lack thereof, retirement).

Having done all this, take a breath and move on to *current* social history. You may need to know about many things, including

- Current living environment
  - Physical location and layout
  - Who lives there
  - Help available, etc.

- Occupation, and how well the job is going in terms of
  - Job performance
  - Interpersonal relationships at work
- Religious or other subcultural or community affiliations
- Current social environment
  - Important people in the patient's life now
  - How much contact the patient has with these persons
  - The qualitative nature of these relationships
  - Socioeconomic conditions
  - Functional abilities (if not already clear from HPI and physical history sections), such as activities of daily living the patient can and can't perform unassisted
  - A sense of the normal daily routine for the patient (if not already apparent from the above)

REVIEW OF SYSTEMS

In addition to the usual thorough "medical" review of systems (ROS)—again, don't sell "psych patients" short on the competency of your evaluation of physical symptoms—use this section to check that you asked about all relevant current and past psychiatric symptoms. It's amazing how often patients avoid spontaneously mentioning obsessions or compulsions, eating disorder behaviors, or nightmares of past sexual abuse, but will answer openly when asked. Obviously, you can't run through the entire *Diagnostic and Statistical Manual of Mental Disorders* (DSM-IV) with each patient, but with experience and knowledge regarding common psychiatric comorbidities, you'll learn what questions constitute a relevant psychiatric ROS for a given patient.

PHYSICAL EXAMINATION

Too often this section of the workup is given short shrift, considering the comorbidity of medical and mental disorders. Along with the general physical examination, pay close attention to a careful screening neurological examination at minimum (and more than that if the medical history, general physical, or cognitive examination suggests the likelihood of neurological disease). For patients with severe mental illnesses, it is especially important to note nonlateralizing neurological findings that are often associated with "primary" as well as secondary psychiatric disorders, and with side effects of psychotropic medication. These may include

- Adventitious movements (dyskinesia, tremors)
- Subtle dysarthrias
- Gait abnormalities

heart murmur, is of pathological concern, not every abnormality on the MSE indicates psychopathology. For example, mild psychomotor slowing could be related to tiredness, or to normal-level anxiety during the interview. On the other hand, it could be related to a depressive or psychotic disorder, or to neuroleptic-induced parkinsonism. The *interpretation* of the slowing depends on the entire clinical context and does not belong in the MSE. In any case, don't neglect mentioning the observation for fear of "pathologizing" the patient.

- Many textbooks suggest writing the MSE in paragraph form. This is fine for experienced MSE-writers, but for trainees, it's probably more useful to write the MSE as a list with the headings as suggested here, analogous to the list of headings you use for the PE ("HEENT, Lungs, Cardiac, etc."). This will help you quickly to get comfortable with the crucial skill of breaking down your behavioral observations into components.

- Too often the term "mental status" is used synonymously with "cognitive status." Think of what's usually meant when you've heard that a patient has "mental status changes," or how many times you've heard someone say they didn't "do" a mental status examination "on" the patient. Remember, the MSE covers a wide range of mental experiences and manifestations, of which cognition is only one part. Most of the MSE can be described by a trained observer (which is what you're here to become) after *any* patient interview.

- Part of the goal of developing your MSE skills is to learn to use the relevant technical jargon properly, with all the advantages of terseness and precision that jargon is supposed to provide. To take another analogy from general medicine, you wouldn't say, "The patient had rales, with a crunchy kind of sound audible through the stethoscope." You would simply say "The patient had rales," perhaps with an adjectival specifier, such as "fine rales" or "coarse wet rales." Yet many trainees initially tend to say the equally redundant, "The patient's thought processes were tangential; he was unable to stick to one subject and tended to drift from one topic to another." Avoid this wordiness (although doing so means you have to learn what the proper jargon is)! On the other hand, adjectival specifiers often are useful (e.g., "mild tangentiality"). Brief examples or other specifics, as will be described in each section, may also be useful.

Let us now dissect the MSE.

GENERAL APPEARANCE AND BEHAVIOR

This and the next section set the stage, as it were, for the rest of the MSE. Among other things, they help convey a sense of how complete and accurate the MSE is likely to be. Things to consider and possibly comment on include:

- What is the patient's level of hygiene and grooming?
- What is the patient's choice of clothing? More than aesthetics is involved here. Is the patient wearing a T-shirt and shorts in snowy weather, a down jacket and ski hat in the summer, sunglasses while inside (this may reflect paranoia or an ophthalmologic

Incongruous dress

condition), garish clashing colors (this may reflect mania or hyperthymic temperament), or a perfectly pressed gray pinstripe three-piece suit (may reflect occupation, socioeconomic status, obsessive personality style, or need to appear successful or important).

- Where is the patient seen? (In bed? While pacing in the hall?)
- Are there any unusual motor activities or mannerisms?
- Does the patient appear his or her age?

QUALITY OF RELATIONSHIP TO INTERVIEWER

The important things here are to comment tersely on the manner in which the patient relates to the interviewer. This may be gauged partly by commenting on the degree of eye contact; descriptors typically including "none," "fair" or "occasional," "good" or "normal," and "excessive" or "intense" or "unwavering." Also, what is the tone of the relationship? Terms to consider here include "warm," "neutral," "reserved," "hostile" or "angry," "guarded," "suspicious," "flirtatious" or "seductive," "withdrawn," or "totally unengaged." These qualities may vary during the interview, and can be described as such: For example, "He was initially hostile, but engaged progressively and well by the interview's end."

PSYCHOMOTOR ACTIVITY

Technically, this section might include all motor behavior observed during the interview. In practice, this section is often used to describe all such activity beyond what has already been described in the motor section of the neurological examination. Thus, in abbreviated reports that do not include a neurological exam, this would be the place to describe evident tremulousness, tics, dyskinesia, akathisia, or choreiform movements. If such movements dominate the overall appearance of the patient, they would be mentioned in the "General Appearance" section as well.

Aside from adventitious movements, this section should describe any other *unusual motor activity*, such as posturing movements of the extremities or waxy flexibility (sustained posturing combined with the potential for passive manipulation of the position). Describe any *motor hypoactivity* (psychomotor retardation), which may manifest in slowness of verbal responses (increased speech latency), actual slowing of movements, or decreased initiation of movements. Also mention any evident *hyperactivity*. This is usually referred to as "psychomotor agitation," but give specifics: There's a lot of difference between the psychomotor agitation of hand wringing and that of pacing with fists clenched. Note that it is possible to have *both* agitation and retardation at the same time. Many severely depressed patients, for example, have overall psychomotor slowing with subtle superimposed agitation (leg rocking, foot tapping, hand wringing).

SPEECH

Different textbooks have varied approaches to this topic. Some include items such as language and thought process, which I've put in other sections for didactic purposes. In the narrow view adopted here, speech encompasses the *physical* production of verbal output. Thus, things to note include:

- Dysphonia (trouble with the production of vocal "wind," e.g., hoarseness, limited volume)
- Dysarthria (trouble with articulation)
- Volume
- Amount (if increased, may be referred to as *logorrhea*)
- Speed
- Modulation and inflection (*dysprosody* is the neurological term for loss of speech melody)
- Spontaneous speech versus responsive speech only
- Latency (see also "Psychomotor Activity")
- Pressured speech (You've got to see and hear this to really understand it, but basically this is a sense of force or pressure behind the words, even beyond the volume, amount, or speed of speech, that makes it hard to interrupt.)

MOOD AND AFFECT

These terms are used to describe the patient's emotional state. They are often referred to as if they were separate, but in practice the distinctions between mood and affect blur and are often ignored. Still, the principle can be seen from an analogy in that dreaded old Scholastic Aptitude Test format, *mood :: affect* as *climate :: weather.* In other words, mood is the overall prevailing emotional state (during the interview, not the Cenozoic era), and affect is the variability of emotions during the course of the interview.

Often mood is determined by asking the patient about it (e.g., "How would you describe your mood, your spirits?"). Quote the patient when possible, but feel free to offer your own assessment if it differs from the patient's verbatim response. For instance, you might write, "Mood—patient states 'fine,' but appears depressed." Words used when describing mood include "neutral," "sad/depressed/down," "happy," "euphoric," "expansive" (meaning euphoric to the max), "anxious" (and its thousand synonyms—"tense," "nervous," "worried," etc.), "irritable" (easily angered), "angry."

For affect, plan on commenting on the following domains:

- Intensity—How *much* emotion is expressed or exuded? If affective intensity is severely reduced, terms such as "flat" or "blunted" are used.
- Range—Is the affect stuck in one position for the whole interview, or does it vary? If it varies, describe how (e.g., "from neutral to tearfulness to mild anger").
- Appropriateness (to thought content)—Does the patient's affect seem congruous with what he or she is talking about?
- Lability—Does the affect shift from one emotion to another with an abnormally rapid, all-or-nothing quality? (Think of turning on a water spigot from off to full pressure in a flash.) If labile affect is present, describe what it is, such as labile tearfulness, labile anger, or labile laughter or euphoria. (Note that in neurological or neuropsychiatric settings, labile affect, especially if inappropriate to content, is often described as "emotional incontinence" or "pseudobulbar affect.")
- Reactivity—Does the affect change appropriately with shifts in thought content, or is it truly unchanging? For example, it is im-

portant to note whether persons with depressed mood can reactively brighten during the course of the interview. (In some texts, reactivity is described as an attribute of mood rather than of affect. You were forewarned that the distinction between mood and affect is useful but somewhat arbitrary.)

THOUGHT CONTENT

As should be apparent, this section is used to describe the content of what's on the patient's mind. In keeping with the concise, focused style of a good MSE, though, don't dwell at great length on all of the patient's worries; that's what the HPI and other previous sections are supposed to do. Rather, highlight in a sentence or so what the prominent themes are, especially if they relate to the presenting problems, for example, nihilistic or guilty themes in a depressed patient, grandiose themes in mania, and so on. Even more important, comment on the presence or absence of "abnormal" thought content, which mostly means:

- Delusions (firmly held beliefs that are falsifiable and not culturally bound)
- Suicidal or homicidal ideation
- Obsessions (see pages 72–73)
- Overvalued ideas (unshakable convictions that are not falsifiable enough to count as delusions, and are not ego-alien enough to count as obsessions)
- Poverty of content (paucity of ideas or topics about which the patient converses, which may be seen in cognitive deficit or depressive disorders)

It helps to give examples or descriptions of any abnormal thought content; for instance, "Persecutory delusions are present, with beliefs that his telephone is being tapped by the FBI," or "He has obsessional thoughts regarding whether or not he killed someone in an automobile accident."

To elicit suicidal ideation (SI), it is helpful to ask about a gradient of self-destructive thoughts, but don't shy away from asking the big question directly, too. For instance, you might ask, "Have you had thoughts that life is not worth living?," followed by "Have you thought about wanting to die, or wanting to take your own life?" In the MSE write-up, SI should encompass descriptions of:

- Ideation
- Plans (Did the patient have a method in mind?)
- Intent (Did the patient get to the point of thinking he or she actually would do it?)

If the patient actually attempted suicide, presumably you've already discussed this in the HPI or Past Psychiatric History sections, as appropriate. Similar issues apply to homicidal ideation, for instance, "Have you ever had thoughts about harming someone else?"

THOUGHT PROCESS

Thought process is concerned with the flow of the patient's ideas and how well they connect with one another. Terms used to describe normal thought process include "logical," "goal-directed," and "well organized." A variety of mildly entertaining terms are used to describe thought process "derailments," or disruptions in goal-directed process:

- *Tangentiality:* literally going off on a tangent; that is, starting on one topic, and in linear fashion straying off the topic until the patient (and the listener) wind up somewhere way out in left field. Mild forms of this may be found in normal persons, but severe forms may indicate psychosis.

- *Circumstantiality:* literally talking around the topic at hand, in such a way that the listener can figure out what the topic is, but the patient isn't able to speak directly and pointedly about the main issue. Again, this may range in severity from normal to psychotic.

- *Thought Blocking:* the patient's train of thought suddenly comes to a halt, and so does his or her verbal output. Of course, it's your job to figure out if the patient stopped talking because of true thought blocking, or for some other reason (e.g., the patient decided not to say what he or she was about to say, or needed a sip of water before proceeding).

- *Loosening of Associations:* in casual conversation among mental health folks, you'll hear expressions such as "that patient was really loose" to refer to any kind of thought-process disturbance. Technically, though, loose associations specifically mean that the patient jumps from topic A to topic D—or even Z—and the listener cannot follow the leap from the first topic to the second.

- *Flight of Ideas:* classically seen in manic syndromes, patients with flight of ideas move rapidly from one topic to another, usually across several topics in a rapid sequence. In pure flight of ideas—i.e., without the commonly superimposed loose associations— the listener can follow each step of the sequence if they can keep up with the patient's pace, but often the patient shifts subjects so rapidly and so frequently that the listener is left baffled, and the patient winds up way off the initial topic.

- *Word Salad:* incoherent speech, technically due to troubled thinking rather than to dysarthria or dysphasia. On the other hand, it may be rather hard to distinguish word salad from a fluent dysphasia, and either may coexist with a dysarthric condition (e.g., from medications).
- *Ruminative Thinking:* the tendency to dwell on the same theme. In its most severe forms, this manifests as the inability to talk about anything other than one topic, despite the interviewer's attempts to shift the subject.
- *Perseveration:* repetition of the same word, short phrase, or syllable. A verbal manifestation of difficulty shifting attention; see the section on "Attention" on pages 146–147.

Other descriptors of thought-process disturbances include *echolalia* (repetitious echoing of words or syllables uttered by the interviewer), *clang associations* (uttering words that rhyme, alliterate, or are otherwise associated by their sound rather than by their sense or meaning), and *punning* (linking phrases only by the use of homonyms, not by their sense). These disturbances are more fascinating than common.

PERCEPTUAL DISTURBANCES

This means just what it says: Describe any abnormalities of perception. These boil down to *hallucinations,* which are sensory perceptions wholly without external basis, and *illusions*, which are gross distortions of actual sensory input. If possible, specify the content of the perceptual disturbance: What did the patient see or hear? Also specify the sensory modality involved: Are the hallucinations auditory (the most common), visual, or (less common) olfactory, tactile, or gustatory? Before documenting the *absence* of hallucinations, be sure to ask the patient directly if he or she has any unusual sensory experiences ("Do you ever hear things that other people don't hear?"). Also, some patients will deny hallucinations, perhaps out of fear or embarrassment, but during the interview may appear to be "responding to internal stimuli." In these cases, describe what you saw, such as "Mr. Xelowicz denied any hallucinations or illusions, but periodically would stop speaking and stare at a corner of the room as if responding to an auditory or visual stimulus."

For the sake of space and simplicity, hallucinations often get lumped together with delusions in many write-ups of the MSE, especially in the negative (e.g., "No delusions or hallucinations"). This practice is probably defensible, as long as you're clear on the conceptual distinction between thought-content (delusions) and sensory disturbances (hallucinations).

COGNITIVE FUNCTIONS

It should be (painfully?) apparent by now that there's far more to the MSE than the cognitive examination. And cognition itself includes a complex, multidimensional range of functions. Cognitive assessments can range from crude screens to fairly detailed "bedside" testing, to extensive, specific, well standardized tasks using pen, paper, blocks, and other prepared materials. The latter is known as neuropsychological testing and requires special training to administer and a doctorate-level psychologist with special training to interpret it properly. For most patients, though, a skilled bedside cognitive examination is sufficient.

At a minimum, you can almost always make some comments about cognition based on any patient interview. The common statement, "I wasn't able to test cognition," often betrays ignorance or laziness regarding cognitive examination. From most interviews, you can describe level of consciousness ("alert"), attentiveness to the interview (not "attention was intact," which implies more formal testing, but "patient was attentive to the interview" or "patient was distractible"), recall of recent or remote events ("memory was not formally tested, but recall of the events leading to admission appeared intact"), language ("language not formally tested, but there were no evident paraphasic errors or other language difficulties during the interview"), and sometimes visuospatial skills ("patient came to my office today for the first time and had no difficulty finding the office by following the map provided").

Such informal cognitive testing is adequate when there is no suspicion of cognitive deficits or altered brain function after review of the history, physical examination, laboratory values, or the remainder of the MSE. However, if there are any doubts regarding these issues—which there should be in all cases of major mental disorder with new onset or unexpected recurrence—then informal observation of cognitive status is complementary to, but is not a substitute for, formal cognitive testing. Also, as a trainee, you are better off gaining experience by attempting to complete a reasonably thorough cognitive examination on all of your patients when possible.

Let me provide an additional friendly warning before proceeding to the details of formal cognitive testing. Most students encounter the Mini-

Mental State Examination (MMSE), a 30-point scale that has been well validated as a screening instrument for cognitive deficits in certain populations. Its usefulness as a screen in acutely ill psychiatric patients is more limited. Even more important, rote application of the MMSE is guaranteed to prevent you from truly understanding the cognitive examination, for several reasons:

- The MMSE emphasizes a *total* score (i.e., 23 out of 30), whereas what counts clinically is knowing what *specific realms* of cognition are impaired.
- Some realms of cognition are poorly covered by the MMSE, which is fine as a brief screening instrument but is a poor substitute for a good cognitive examination.
- On the MMSE, the patient loses points for wrong answers no matter how close or far off a response is, yet clinically it matters a great deal if the patient is off by a little or a lot (e.g., being off on the date by 1 day versus thinking the year is now 1927).

So feel free to familiarize yourself with the MMSE if you encounter it, but don't think that knowing it alone means you've mastered the cognitive examination. Let us now consider the specific components of the cognitive examination.

Level of Consciousness

Level of consciousness (LOC) exists on a continuum. A normal level of wakefulness is described as "alert." There are "hyperalert/hypervigilant" states, which are documented as such. "Lethargy" does not mean lazy, anergic, or slothful when used in a medical/psychiatric context. Rather, lethargy is used to denote a decreased

LOC (i.e., drowsiness), from which the patient can be aroused easily, although relapse is rapid after the arousing stimulus subsides. Furthest down the continuum is *coma,* a state of unarousable, unresponsive unconsciousness. In between lethargy and coma, descriptors such as "obtundation" and "stupor" are often used, although the lack of precise boundaries makes terse narrative descriptions more useful (e.g., "Mr. Pompey was unresponsive to verbal or light touch stimulation. To sternal pressure, he responded with a brief moan and purposeless motions of his upper extremities.").

Orientation

Orientation is, after LOC, the most common cognitive examination documented in patient charts. At times, this documentation may be done erroneously: Don't ever make the mistake of writing "oriented × 3" unless you formally assess all three spheres. Orientation is genuinely useful as a quick and dirty (well, maybe not dirty) screen for cognition, because orientation is actually not a single, fundamental cognitive function. Rather, to remain oriented one must rely on several cognitive capacities, including adequate LOC, language skills, memory, attention to environmental cues, and so on. So orientation is not terribly specific, but its sensitivity makes it useful.

The three spheres of the "× 3" are *person, place,* and *time.* It's important to specify what was tested in each case. For *person,* did you assess orientation to self? To the interviewer's name or role? To other people? In each case, if the patient was incorrect, document what he or she said to help clarify the level of impairment. For example, if the patient met you for the first time yesterday, and today was unable to recall your name, but did know your role ("you're my student doctor"), this is a degree of "disorientation" that often would be considered within normal range, unlike an insistence that you have come to fix the television set. For *place*, things to assess and document include state, city, county, hospital name (if you're in the hospital at the time!), floor, and part of the hospital (emergency room, psychiatry ward). For *time*, it is important to ask about day of the week as well as date, because most healthy persons will remember the day more accurately than the exact date. You also can ask about the month, season, and year. Again, don't just document "disoriented to time": What precisely was the patient's response? If the patient answered, "I don't know," did he or she seem to expend some effort on the task, or does the "I don't know" really reflect "I don't want to try?"

Also, if the patient has difficulty with orientation responses, you might try multiple-choice cues to see if he or she can pull out the correct answers. Tips on cueing are found on pages 147–148, under "Memory."

Attention

The concept of attention is indistinguishably tied to that of *concentration*, although patients' subjective reports of their ability to concentrate may be quite different from their actual performance on formal tests of attention. Also, attention may be impaired in two ways. First, people may have difficulty *shifting* their attention from one task to the next. They consequently tend to get stuck on the first task; such "stickiness" is known as *perseveration*. Perseveration may be evident during many parts of the mental status examination. For example, you ask the patient's age and he or she responds "64"; then you ask the year and the patient says "1964." This is an example of verbal perseveration. Or, while testing constructional abilities (see below), the patient might copy a circle correctly, then draw a circle again when asked to copy a square; this is an example of perseveration on a visuomotor task. Other ways of testing for perseveration are described under "Frontal Executive Functions" on pages 151–152.

The second way in which attention may be impaired, and the more common thing to test, is trouble *sustaining* attention on a task. In severe forms, gross distractibility may be evident during the interview. Formal tests may elicit subtle troubles with sustained attention. You've probably asked patients to perform "serial 7s," that is, to subtract 7 serially from 100. This is supposed to test attention, but of course it also depends on being able to do the arithmetic. Spelling "world" backwards is another common test of sustained attention, but again it helps to know if the patient can spell "world" forward first. Other tests of sustained attention include digit span (how many digits can the patient repeat forward or backward), and the "A" Random Letter Test (known to most simply as the "A" test), in which you intone a steady slow stream of random letters and ask the patient to raise his or her hand or otherwise indicate every time he or she hears the letter "A."

Memory

Memory is a complex realm of functions, as indicated by attempts to distinguish subtypes: immediate, short-term, or long-term memory, or verbal and nonverbal memory. The most common bedside test of memory is asking patients to repeat the names of three objects (*registration*), and then asking them to recall the objects after 5 minutes of doing something else (usually other parts of the cognitive examination). It is helpful to document more than simply how many of the three objects the patient spontaneously remembers at 5 minutes (*free recall*). Can he or she remember any more of the objects if given an abstract clue, known as a *categorical cue*? (Example: if the object was "apple," say, "It was a kind of fruit; now can you remember what it was?") If categorical cueing doesn't work, then try multiple choice or *word list cueing* (e.g., "Was it a pear, apple, or banana?") Your documentation might read as follows: "Pt. registered 3 objects easily, recalled 1/3 at 5 minutes, 2/3 with categorical and 3/3 with word list cues." The point of all this cueing is to distinguish between trouble *retrieving* a memory (which cueing can aid) and *storing* the memory in the first place (which, if impaired, won't be helped by all the cueing in the world).

Bedside tests of long-term memory include asking about recent or remote events, but it is important that you have some way of confirming that the patient's memories are accurate! Aside from recall of the HPI, ask the patient about some major news events or themes of the day, trying to choose a widely known topic or one that you'd expect this particular patient to know. For example, if the patient has reported being a major pro basketball fan, then ask about current league standings or player performances—*if* you know the answers yourself. For testing more remote memory, ask about the overlearned details that most persons should know about themselves, such as birth date, wedding date, names of their siblings or children, and so on. You also can ask what they recall about major news events of past years. Most Americans over the age of 65 years should be able to tell you about Pearl Harbor, and most Americans over the age of 45 years should be able to tell you the place and circumstances of President Kennedy's assassination.

Language

Pay attention to the patient's *vocabulary*. Is the range and use of words appropriate to his or her level of education? Does the patient have *word-finding* troubles? Does he or she make *paraphasic* errors? Test for *dysnomic dysphasia* by asking the patient to name objects, perhaps starting with the commonly used "pen" and "watch." If needed, move on to subtler naming, such as parts of the watch (band, buckle, minute hand, stem or winder, etc.). If the patient can't name the object but tells you what it does, this is an *in*correct response known as a *circumlocutory error*. Test for *repetition dysphasia* by having the patient repeat phrases comprised of short syllables, such as "no ifs, ands, or buts," or "Methodist Episcopal." Test for *verbal fluency* by asking him or her to name as many words that start with "d" as possible in 1 minute, or as many things as he or she can think of that might be found in a grocery store.

Fund of Knowledge

Although all tests of cognition are affected by intelligence, education, and cultural background, fund of knowledge is one of the most severely so, making it tough to interpret difficulties of this kind in some patients. Asking about current or past world events, as per the section on memory above, isn't a bad way to start. Texts on MSE have examples of other things to ask, which at times may be of use (e.g., "Where does rain come from?").

Visuospatial Skills

Visuospatial skills are usually tested by a variety of pencil-and-paper tasks. Common tests include asking the patient to copy figures (e.g., a circle, a square, intersecting pentagons, a rendering of a cube), to draw a clock (instructions to put the hands at "10:10" makes the task more difficult, and therefore more sensitive to deficits), or to draw a floor plan of his or her home. It is most helpful to place the patient's actual attempts in the chart, rather than simply stating "unable" in the write-up.

Less formal, more "conversational" assessment of visuospatial skills is difficult, but may be addressed partially by asking ambulatory patients to find their rooms (or some other nearby destination), or nonambulatory patients to describe how they would get to such a destination. These techniques are, of course, considerably confounded by memory impairments.

Calculations

Arithmetic skills, while clearly affected by education and native intelligence, may be impaired specifically in various cognitive deficit disorders. Ask the patient to perform one-step operations: "How much is 15 plus 17? What is 4 times 6?" and so on. Make the problems simpler if necessary. Alternatively, you can ask the patient to perform tasks involving making monetary change: "If you had a dollar and bought a newspaper for 25 cents, how much change would you get?"

Frontal Executive Functions

Frontal executive functions (FEFs) are probably the least tangible and hardest to describe of the cognitive functions. Basically, in order to function in our daily lives, we need to organize, prioritize, sequence, and execute a variety of mental and physical actions. In doing so, we draw on memory, language, and the other cognitive realms, but the processes of *organizing* and *sequencing* are themselves liable to impairment. Patients with diseases affecting frontal lobe structure and function may demonstrate such difficulties, hence the origin of the term "frontal executive functions." Deficits in FEFs may have enormous implications for a patient's ability to negotiate life in the real world.

The MMSE includes a simple, crude FEF test—the three-step command, "Take the paper in your right hand, fold it in half, and put it in your lap." Other approaches to FEFs recognize that part of FEFs involves shifting attention when necessary, which overlaps with the concept of perseveration discussed earlier. One way to test for motor perseveration at the bedside is to ask the patient to copy this diagram:

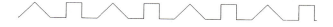

If the patient makes errors of repeating the same component, as shown below, the deficit is termed "graphomotor perseveration":

↑

Perseverative Error

A second test is to ask patients to perform three motions with one hand sequentially: "pound" the table (or their knee) once with a fist, then "cut" the table once with fingers outstretched and hand held vertically, and finally "pat" the table once with fingers outstretched but hand held prone. Have patients repeat this sequence—fist, edge, palm—as rapidly as they can, first with one hand and then with the other. Observe for slowness, perseverative errors (e.g., fist twice before edge), and sequence errors (e.g., fist, palm, edge). Any errors that cannot be accounted for by simple motor weakness may be ascribed to frontal lobe dysfunction on the contralateral side.

There are lots of other tests for FEFs that require prepared materials to administer. Check a neuropsychology reference, or consult your nearest friendly neuropsychologist, if you're curious or have a patient needing more extensive evaluation in this area.

Abstraction

"Rarely have so many spent so much effort on so little." This somewhat hyperbolic paraphrase of Churchill is intended to serve as a caution in testing and interpreting abstraction, the ability to move from concrete symbolism to broader, generalizable intellectual constructs. There are plenty of problems in testing this ability:

- A substantial portion of the adult population, by dint of intelligence, education, and perhaps lots of other things, functions at a fairly concrete level. In other words, if your patient answers your tests of abstraction concretely, don't automatically assume that this represents a decline from baseline. On the other hand, if a person with a PhD in philosophy is unable to abstract, something must be going on. (How's that for an abstract conclusion?)

- Most students dutifully test abstraction as they were taught, namely, by asking for proverb interpretation. Yet this adds further layers of difficulty in interpreting the results, as proverb interpretation may be heavily influenced by cultural background and by whether or not the patient has heard this particular proverb before.

Given these problems, it is probably more useful to test abstraction by asking the patient about similarities. Begin by giving the patient an example of what you're after. "Ms. Ventana, I'd like you to tell me how the following things are similar, or what they have in common. For instance, if I asked you what was similar about a car and a boat, you might say that they're both means of transportation. Now, how are an apple and a banana similar?" If Ms. Ventana replies "They're both fruits," she gets credit for an abstract response. If she says, "They both have skin," she has answered correctly but concretely. If she says, "They're both red," she has given a wrong response. If she says, "They're both offspring of the earth, and part of Nature's grand plan," then her response is hyperabstract and suggests the possibility of associated expansive mood.

Other bedside tests of abstraction ask about differences. For example, "Which of the following does not belong with the others—a boy, a door, or a man?"

JUDGMENT AND INSIGHT

Judgment refers in a general way to the ability to plan and act wisely and in accord with established cultural norms. Some texts suggest assessing judgment by asking the patient what he or she would do in certain circumstances: "What would you do if you smelled smoke in a movie theater?" With acutely ill patients, it is often more useful to assess judgment based on the patient's recent actions leading to clinical presentation. For example, a patient brought to the emergency department by the police, having been found wandering outside in subzero temperatures wearing only shorts and a T-shirt, has evidenced poor judgment, regardless of how well he or she responds to a question about smoke in the theater.

Insight refers to accuracy and depth of understanding of a situation. In clinical contexts, the situation that usually matters most is insight into the patient's own illness or troubles. How well does the patient's understanding of the illness jibe with yours or with what the patient has been told by previous treating physicians? Does the patient accept that anything in his or her behavior is wrong, or does he or she externalize all blame on others? How does the patient respond when you explain (in language appropriate to the clinical state) your assessment of the psychiatric condition or need for treatment?

13
CHAPTER

Laboratory Evaluations and Psychological Testing

PLANNING A LABORATORY WORKUP

As described in Chapter 4, the range of medical and neurological conditions that may contribute to psychopathology includes most of the rest of medicine. Given this, it's rather hard to list all the laboratory procedures that might be used in the psychiatric workup. Adding to the difficulty of making such a list useful is the need for clinical judgment, including benefit/cost considerations, in each specific case.

So let us just try to give a few general guidelines:

- Most important—and I hope most obvious—are direct clues from the patient's current symptoms, medical history, and physical examination. These may lead directly to specific laboratory tests that might not be necessary otherwise. For example, for a healthy 35-year-old man with new-onset major depression of moderate severity, a reasonable laboratory workup would initially be limited to some basic screening blood tests (complete blood count, electrolyte and glucose levels, etc.). But if the same patient were known to have human immunodeficiency virus (HIV)–seropositivity, he would require extensive laboratory evaluation, beginning with a larger panel of blood work, probably a neuroimaging study such as a computed tomography or magnetic resonance imaging scan, and possibly a lumbar puncture.

- Patients presenting with cognitive deficit disorders (e.g., delirium, dementia) by implication and by definition have one or more "organic" contributors to their condition. The workup to delineate these contributors must be thorough, as discussed in Chapter 4.

- If your patient does not have specific worrisome features from the medical history and evaluation and does not have a cognitive deficit syndrome, then use the following clinical criteria as guidelines to suggest the need for laboratory evaluation beyond that required for normal health maintenance:

  - *Any* new-onset psychiatric syndrome in an elderly person, including mood, psychotic, anxiety, or somatoform syndromes
  - New-onset mania or psychosis in a person of any age
  - New-onset anxiety or somatoform syndromes in a person older than say, 30 years who lacks prior psychiatric history and also lacks evidence for personality disorder
  - Clear, sustained "personality" change in the absence of an idiopathic Axis I disorder that could account for the change

- Syndromes that fail to respond to adequate treatment (e.g., a 25-year-old moderately depressed woman who shows no improvement after adequate trials of one or two antidepressant medications)
- Recurrence of a known psychiatric condition that is not consistent with its prior course in that patient, and is not explainable by medication noncompliance, new psychosocial stressors, or other circumstances

In each of these scenarios, the exact nature of the laboratory workup required will depend on demographic and clinical details, standards of practice in a given community, and cost/benefit analyses.

TYPES OF PSYCHOLOGICAL TESTING

"Psychological testing" refers to a broad array of tests administered by trained personnel, employing interview, pen and paper, or other means. Doctorate-level psychologists are particularly qualified to administer and interpret the results of these tests. Briefly, types of testing may include:

- *Intelligence Testing.* These tests measure global intellectual function, although subscores may focus on particular realms (e.g., "Verbal Intelligence Quotient"). They are normed to the general population by age, with "100" being average. Specific scores have been used to define various levels of mental retardation or superior function ("genius").

- *Neuropsychological Testing.* As mentioned previously, these are tests designed to assess performance in specific cognitive realms. As such, they may complement bedside cognitive testing and may serve to document stability or changes in cognition over time.
- *Personality Testing.* These are typically pen-and-paper tests that depend on self-reported responses to questions assessing a variety of aspects of personality style and traits. Of course, current state of mind can influence the ways in which patients respond. These tests are of considerable use in clinical research and have applicability to vocational assessments and other applied psychology settings. Their usefulness is limited in most psychiatric settings, especially in those caring for acutely ill patients.
- *Projective Testing.* These tests ask patients to respond in an open-ended and expansive manner to standardized stimuli such as inkblots (Rorschach) or drawings of evocative scenes (e.g., Thematic Apperception Test). Psychologists trained to "score" these unstructured responses in structured ways interpret the results, yielding information on themes, conflicts, and affects prominent in the patient's mental life (but often not obvious from clinical interviews of similar length). Projective testing is not a substitute for diagnosis based on clinical evaluation of symptoms, but it may aid the diagnostic process by revealing psychotic thought processes, depressive themes, or other aspects that are not clearly evident otherwise.

14
CHAPTER

Diagnostic Impression, Formulation, and Plan

Every psychiatric workup will end with some kind of summation (to carry the previous legal analogy to its inexorable conclusion). This summation will basically convey what you *think* about the data you've just gathered, organized, and presented, and also what you plan to *do* from here. A commonly used format includes:

- Diagnostic impression (essentially a list of diagnoses)
- Formulation (an opportunity to discuss differential diagnostic thinking, or to consider etiologic issues)
- Plan (a description of what you're going to do)

The lengths of these sections, particularly the latter two, may vary enormously depending on the clinical setting. For example, a workup of an inpatient with a first psychotic presentation probably should have a formulation section that considers the differential diagnosis and etiologic contributors in some detail. By contrast, an emergency room workup of a patient already diagnosed and well established in outpatient treatment is likely to be much shorter and will focus on the presenting crisis and intervention plans rather than on formulation.

Also, as a trainee you may be asked to write more complete "summations" than would be needed otherwise, presumably to further your learning and allow you to demonstrate to your teachers what you know and how you think about the clinical problems at hand. So it is important for you to ask your preceptors about their expectations.

RECORDING YOUR
DIAGNOSTIC IMPRESSION

To begin with, you will probably be asked to put your diagnostic impression in the style of the *Diagnostic and Statistical Manual of Mental Disorder* (DSM-IV) multiaxial format, as listed in Table 14–1. Following are some thoughts about what to include for each axis:

Axis I: Most psychiatric diagnoses go here. So do the DSM-IV "V Codes," that is, important conditions that don't count as true mental disorders (e.g., normal bereavement). Be sure to include rule-outs, or "X vs. Y," if the diagnosis is unclear, but try to indicate what you think is *most* likely (example in Table 14–2). Also be sure to include all diagnoses here (e.g., chronic schizophrenia AND cocaine dependence).

Axis II: Again, include rule-outs when applicable. Personality disorder diagnosis may be deferred if available data are too scant to suggest the presence or absence of one, but if

Table 14–1. MULTIAXIAL ASSESSMENT

AXIS	WHAT IT COVERS
Axis I	Clinical disorders Other conditions that may be a focus of clinical attention
Axis II	Personality disorders Mental retardation
Axis III	General medical conditions
Axis IV	Psychosocial and environmental problems
Axis V	Global assessment of functioning

Source: Adapted from American Psychiatric Association: Diagnostic and Statistical Manual of Mental Disorders, 4th ed. Washington, DC, American Psychiatric Association, 1994, p 25, with permission.

the data point to the likelihood that personality pathology is or isn't present, say so!

Axis III: This list of medical illnesses should include rule-outs or differentials when appropriate. Be sure to include the diagnoses that cause any cognitive or secondary disorders on Axis I.

Axis IV: This axis should record any stressful life events, usually referred to as *stressors,* or ongoing problematic environmental issues ("environment" meaning the patient's psychosocial milieu).

Axis V: Place a number from 0 to 100 here, reflecting your estimate of the patient's level of functioning on the Global Assessment of Functioning (GAF) scale in DSM-IV. It's often useful to score both the patient's *current* GAF and *baseline* GAF (e.g., highest func-

Table 14–2. SAMPLE MULTIAXIAL ASSESSMENT

Axis I	Major depressive disorder vs. alcohol-induced mood disorder, depressed type vs. mood disorder due to antihypertensive medications Alcohol dependence R/O social phobia
Axis II	R/O avoidant personality disorder
Axis III	Asthma, stable Essential hypertension
Axis IV	Separation from spouse Decrease in income d/t job layoff
Axis V	Current GAF 35–40 High GAF in past year 65–70

tioning in the last year). Rate disability caused solely by psychiatric issues, not physical limitations. Note that almost all patients sick enough to require inpatient care will have GAF scores less than 40. Many persons with personality disorders or other chronic psychiatric illnesses may score no higher than the 50s on the GAF even when functioning at their best.

RECORDING YOUR FORMULATION

As you move on to write your formulation, keep the following things in mind.

First, discuss the DSM-IV diagnoses. That is, how do the patient's symptoms cluster together into recognizable *syndromes*? How do these syndromes fit into particular disorders? For example, defend why you think a psychotic syndrome is caused by medication toxicity rather than a primary psychotic disorder, or explain why you believe prominent anxiety symptoms are part of a major depressive illness rather than a primary anxiety disorder. Also, if the diagnoses are unclear, what specific data do you need to clarify them? Observation of symptoms over time? Recent observations by other informants? Old records describing previous episodes?

Next, what is the focal problem? In other words, why is the patient presenting *now*? Focal problems that lead to inpatient admission usually involve suicidal ideation, homicidal ideation, or severe functional incapacity. Focal problems for new outpatient presentations may include these and also may include other specific target symptoms ("I'm feeling depressed") or behaviors ("My wife and I are arguing too much"). Ongoing cases, particularly long-term psychotherapy or outpatient management of chronic disorders, may be more difficult to reduce to a single focal problem. But it is still important to identify and prioritize the most important problems and associated short-term and long-term goals of treatment.

Finally, how do you *understand* the patient's diagnoses and focal problem? To answer this, you may choose to consider any or several of the following:

- If there is more than one diagnosis, how do they influence each other?
- How is the focal problem tied to the psychiatric diagnoses?
- How are the focal problem and psychiatric diagnoses related to, or explainable by:
  - Current psychosocial factors such as family dynamics or stressful life events?

- The psychodynamic formulation of the patient—an appraisal of his or her salient conflicts, usual defense mechanisms, and interpersonal relatedness, along with analysis of how these may or may not be related to the current presentation and treatment implementation; this may include a developmental perspective on current psychodynamic issues
- Other psychological perspectives—learning theory, cognitive psychology, etc.
- Genetic factors
- Neurobiologic alterations or mechanisms
- General medical conditions, medications, and other physiological factors
- The mechanisms by which treatments may help the presenting problems

RECORDING YOUR PLAN

The next section should describe your plans. Organize the plans by a problem list, just as you have done in general medical settings. The patient's psychiatric presentation may be encompassed under one item in some cases, or it may be more usefully conceptualized via several different items, especially in patients with multiple diagnoses or complex psychosocial issues (e.g., "family discord" or "social isolation" might be listed as separate problems to be addressed). Don't forget to list and address all medical problems as well. For each problem, describe *what* you will do, and with what *aim*: "Begin nortriptyline to target major depressive syndrome," or "Address cognitive depressive distortions in cognitive/psychoeducational individual psychotherapy," or "Family meeting to discuss psychoeducation, sources of conflict with patient, and resources available after discharge from hospital."

The problem/plan list should end with discussion about overall expectations for the course of treatment. For instance, in the case of inpatient or partial hospital admissions, what is the estimated length of stay, and what is the expected disposition plan? In the case of a new outpatient, how often and how long will the patient be seen, and how will the end of treatment be determined?

4
PART

Psychiatric Treatments

"'Can't seem to talk about the things that bother me,' seems to be what everybody has."
—**The Music Machine,** *Talk Talk,* 1966
(Written by **Sean Bonniwell**)

"They gave me a medicated lotion, but it didn't SOOTHE my emotion!"
—**Ray Charles,** *I Don't Need No Doctor,* 1966
(Written by **Nicholas Ashford and Valerie Simpson**)

Despite the above laments, talking and medication are still the mainstays of psychiatric treatments. There are a few other "somatic" therapies in psychiatry, including electroconvulsive therapy and light therapy. The next couple of chapters will help you ingest the basics of these approaches in two fair-sized gulps.

15

CHAPTER

Psychotherapies

In the narrow—and most commonly used—sense of the term, "psychotherapy" refers to a well-defined form of treatment. Before we consider different types of such specific psychotherapy, though, we should recognize that, in the broadest sense, "psychotherapy" refers to the beneficial effects for the patient of the relationship with the physician or other health care provider. Therefore, all clinicians essentially use "psychotherapy," although usually neither they nor their patients explicitly call it such. It is important to remember that all treatments and other interventions—medications, diagnostic or therapeutic procedures, surgery—depend on and occur within the context of the doctor-patient alliance. After all, few people will take an expensive medicine that causes side effects or allow themselves to be subjected to the discomforts of surgical procedures unless they feel secure enough in the relationship with the doctor to believe that what the doctor offers or recommends is worth the effort. Thus, maintaining a strong, positive therapeutic alliance must be a goal for all clinicians, regardless of specialty.

Also, several aspects of a positive alliance are

therapeutic in and of themselves; that is, they help patients feel better. Being conscious of these aspects in your interactions with patients will help you refine your interpersonal techniques to foster the development and maintenance of positive alliances. Therapeutic factors in the doctor-patient relationship may include:

- *Empathy.* Simply put, patients feel better when they feel emotionally connected to the physician. "Connected to" includes a feeling of being understood, as well as a sense of being cared about and for, all of which are implied by the term "empathy." Physicians can use a number of techniques in the interview to communicate empathy, as you learned in your course work on basic interviewing skills.
- *Role Modeling.* Patients can feel reassured, calmed, or otherwise soothed by the example of the physician's demeanor, assuming that enough alliance is present to make the physician's example meaningful to the patient. (In other words, if the physician is calm but gives the impression of lack of concern for the patient, the patient is unlikely to feel reassured by the physician's calmness!) The physician's attitude of realistic hopefulness may help to engender a sense of hope in the patient. Similarly, patients may usefully adopt their physician's expressed worry about a particular problem, leading to improved compliance with recommended interventions.
- *Direct Reassurance.* Often physicians must reassure patients by words as well as by demeanor. It is critical to maintain empathy while doing so, to ensure that telling the patient that a symptom is not serious does not convey a sense of derision or condescension about the patient's worry. Indeed, one of the

subtlest and most useful interview skills is the ability to communicate—taking the patient's *concern* seriously, even though the patient's *symptom* does not worry you.

- *Education.* One of the basic tasks facing you as a physician is to tell the patient what you think. That is, you must tell the patient how you understand what he or she has, and why you're recommending whatever you're recommending. The nuances of this task involve variations in vocabulary and language style, as well as *what* (i.e., how much) to say *when* (i.e., timing). The "when" also might include *who,* that is, deciding whether or when to include family members or other persons in the discussions. Education is a useful technique for two broad reasons. First, the *content* communicated is important, enabling patients to know enough to join with you in making needed decisions about interventions. Second, the *process* of education (if done properly) fosters both empathy and role modeling, by expressing in action, if not in so many words, your belief that the two of you are working together to address the patient's concerns.

- *Acknowledging Ignorance.* Often you will not be certain about diagnosis, prognosis, or other things. In such situations, you must be explicit and clear with your patient as to what you do and don't know. You also should convey how important or possible you think such certainty is, as well as what you suggest doing next to arrive at any needed clarity. This latter point makes for a smooth segue to . . .

- *Recommendations.* Virtually every patient contact should include some component of recommendations. Many times the recommendation is to do nothing, or to continue the present course of action without change.

Even in these situations, making this explicit to the patient can be enormously reassuring and also can help ensure that in fact nothing different is done. Other times, the recommendation is to await results of a test or procedure, or to observe the course of a symptom over time. Often recommendations have two or more components. For instance, you might say, "Odds are good that your symptoms will gradually resolve over the next 1 to 2 weeks, in which case continue the symptomatic treatments you're already using. If the symptoms don't improve, or if you develop a fever, call me and we'll need to reevaluate at that time." Note how education and recommendations coexist in this statement. This is frequently the case, particularly when recommending a medication or procedure that requires education regarding benefits, potential adverse effects, and so forth. Indeed, careful attention to maintaining the treatment alliance by use of education, empathy, and so on will maximize the likelihood that your patient will follow your recommendations—or, if he or she chooses not to follow them, that this choice can be openly discussed, preserving the possibility of finding alternatives and maintaining a healthy alliance.

These therapeutic factors apply to all patient-clinician encounters. However, mental health professionals and other health care providers may offer more formal psychotherapy as part of the treatment, or the sole treatment, for a variety of mental disorders and emotional conditions. What makes such psychotherapy "more formal" is variable and even somewhat arbitrary. Part of what makes it *Psychotherapy* with a capital "P" is the referral process or other explicit acknowledgment that the talking itself is intended to be therapeutic. This explicitness flows naturally from explanation of treatment goals and methods, since the goals usually involve amelioration of troublesome feelings or patterns of actions. In other words, labeling the process "psychotherapy" (regardless of the actual words) is part of the education and recommendations techniques discussed above. By contrast, in most non–"psychotherapy" doctor-patient encounters, the therapeutic value of the alliance is left unspoken or implied, or is obliquely referred to as the doctor's "bedside manner."

Still, a large part of the technique and effectiveness of most psychotherapies stems from the basic, nonspecific components of the therapeutic alliance discussed above. The more specific techniques of particular psychotherapeutic modalities depend on the supporting framework of a stable, trusting alliance, just as does the use of medications or procedures in medicine and psychiatry.

Neither space nor the intended purpose of this book allows us to consider the detailed practice of any single psychotherapy, let alone the breadth of available psychotherapies. In a manner analogous to our earlier guided tour through various theoretical orientations, let us survey some of the most common psychotherapy styles and their clinical applications.

THE SUPPORTIVE-EXPRESSIVE CONTINUUM

Psychodynamic psychotherapies are, unsurprisingly, based on the psychodynamic principles briefly discussed in Chapter 3. There are two broad types, *supportive* and *expressive,* as described in the next sections. However, while separate sections are a convenient way to convey the differing essences of these approaches, in actual practice, skilled psychodynamic psychotherapists must be flexible enough not to be limited by somewhat arbitrary boundaries. It is probably more useful to consider supportive and expressive psychotherapies as two ends of a spectrum of psychodynamic psychotherapies. The therapist must choose where to be on the spectrum at any given time with a particular patient. Some patients' therapies will be clearly at one end or the other of the spectrum. Many others will be somewhere in between, employing a mixture of supportive and expressive techniques. And many therapies will, in fact, shift along the spectrum during the course of the therapy. They may move closer to the supportive end during times of crisis or symptomatic exacerbation. They may come closer to the expressive end during times of relative stability or after a firm treatment alliance is formed with a predominantly supportive approach. Keep this sense of the potential for flexibility in mind as you read the next two sections.

Indeed, keep a sense of flexibility in mind as you read *all* of the following sections. Although it may be harder to consider, say, psychodynamic and behavioral therapies as a "continuum," in practice many therapists usefully employ a mixture of psychodynamic, behavioral, or cognitive approaches, as well as a mixture of individual, family, or group modalities.

Supportive Psychotherapy

In supportive psychotherapy, the therapist formulates the patient in psychodynamic terms (as one part of the overall psychiatric formulation). Specifically, the therapist notes problematic intrapsychic and interpersonal patterns and—in collaboration with the patient—uses this framework to identify goals for the psychotherapy. The most prominent techniques employed are the nonspecific skills described above, particularly empathic listening, role modeling, education, and recommendations, all in the service of maintaining a positive therapeutic alliance along with achieving the patient-specific goals.

Given this definition, it might seem that supportive psychotherapy is simply "being there," a task that anyone could accomplish. However, it takes great skill to maintain a positive alliance with many patients. Patients may become angry, disappointed, withdrawn, or more overtly "act out" by noncompliance or other self-destructive behaviors during the course of the therapy. The therapist uses psychodynamic understanding to shape responses to such disruptions in the alliance. But although the therapist's notions of unconscious processes, including transference and the relationship of earlier developmental events to current patterns, are crucial to his or her formulation of the patient, only rarely are direct interpretations of unconscious mental processes offered to the patient. Most of the therapist's comments to the patient take the form of questioning, clarifications, confrontations (regarding overtly manifest thoughts and behaviors), and suggestions. The ratio of use of these different types of comments varies greatly depending on the clinical situation. For example, long-term psychotherapy with a poorly functioning schizophrenic patient might include frequent and repeated direct suggestions and opinions about things ranging from the need to take medications to the details of how to go about applying for housing or employment. By contrast, supportive psychotherapy with a patient with a mild personality disorder might include more confrontational comments and fewer direct recommendations to foster patient autonomy and a sense of responsibility for his or her own actions.

Supportive psychotherapy sessions may be as brief as 15 minutes or as long as 1 hour. Sessions are often held weekly. More than one session per week may be needed if the patient is clinically tenuous or in a situation-related crisis. Sessions also may be held less often than weekly, particularly with chronically ill patients whose illnesses and relationships with their therapist are stable.

When is supportive psychotherapy indicated? A partial guide is as follows:

- *Crises.* At times of symptomatic exacerbation or regressed functioning in patients with a wide variety of psychiatric disorders, supportive approaches are generally used to help the patient regain psychic equilibrium.
- *Long-Term Therapy with the Severely Ill.* Patients with chronic mental illnesses, particularly psychotic disorders or more severe variants of mood or personality disorders, are unlikely to benefit from, and may become worse with, attempts at expressive psychotherapy. Supportive psychotherapy is often used, typically in combination with medications or psychosocial interventions (e.g., case management, enriched housing, day programs). Treatment goals may include psychoeducation, treatment compliance, successful negotiation of stressful events, and progress toward other specified goals, such as obtaining or maintaining a job or developing more friends or other social supports.
- *Other Settings.* Supportive approaches may be used in clinical settings not covered by the above categories when (a) specific goals exist for treatment with psychotherapy

(corollary: you don't do *any* psychotherapy unless there's a reason); (b) there are no indications for behavioral, cognitive, or other specific psychotherapies; and (c) expressive psychotherapy is unlikely to be effective or tolerated (see below).

Expressive Psychotherapy

Expressive psychotherapy is often referred to as "insight-oriented" therapy. Like supportive psychotherapy, it is based on psychodynamic theories, but its techniques are much closer to those of traditional psychoanalysis, which is discussed in the next section. Specifically, direct suggestions or recommendations to the patient are kept to a minimum. Rather, the emphasis is on interpretations of behavior, as related to current unconscious mental processes, as well as to developmental issues and their relationship to current mental functioning. Direct interpretations of the transference, particularly negative transference, are also used. These interpretations lead to insight. In other words, the patient comes to understand both the *what* and the *why* of troublesome thoughts, feelings, or actions, which helps him or her to make needed changes.

It should be noted that obtaining such insight is not easy. Unconscious mental processes are usually unconscious for reasons, so the patient may demonstrate *resistance* to interpretations or to the overall therapy. Successful expressive therapy depends on a positive transference—that is, on a therapeutic alliance directly analogous to that of supportive psychotherapy (and of any successful doctor-patient relationship)—which provides the framework for working through any resistance.

It is difficult to accomplish treatment goals with expressive psychotherapy unless sessions are held at least weekly. Some patients may be seen two or three times a week, either (a) to help manage crises or symptomatic exacerbations (in which case the tenor of the therapy may temporarily move more toward the supportive end of the continuum), or (b) to help overcome resistance and otherwise accelerate the pace of insight and clinical improvement.

Expressive psychotherapy may be useful in the following conditions:

- *Relatively mild personality disorders* (or personality-related difficulties that may not even be severe enough to warrant a diagnosis of "disorder"; in these milder cases, the psychotherapy may be used to treat symptoms or to aid "personal growth")
- *Less severe Axis I conditions* such as mild mood or anxiety disorders, particularly when superimposed on personality difficulties

Apart from diagnosis, the following clinical characteristics favor the use of expressive psychotherapy. Their absence suggests that the patient will not benefit from, or tolerate, such treatment:

- Motivation for change
- Psychological mindedness, that is, the ability to observe one's own internal state (introspection) and to make sense of personal observations in psychological terms
- Ability to form a therapeutic alliance as demonstrated by previous successful intimate relationships, capacity to tolerate one's own negative affects, and a reasonable degree of impulse control

PSYCHOANALYSIS

"Pure" psychoanalysis makes up a small percentage of psychotherapies administered in the broad spectrum of clinical practices. Psychoanalysts may be psychiatrists, psychologists, or "lay" analysts, but all have undergone extensive training at psychoanalytic institutes. Psychoanalysis involves four or five hour-long sessions per week, typically extending for several years. The patient is encouraged to express freely all thoughts and associations that come to mind during sessions. To facilitate this process, and to maximize the intensity of transference reactions, the patient usually reclines on a couch while the therapist sits out of the patient's visual field. The analyst makes extensive use of interpretations, both in the "here and now" (e.g., transference interpretations) and as related to developmental issues and earlier life events. In effect, psychoanalysis is an extremely intensified version of expressive psychotherapy. (Historically, the reverse is true: Face-to-face expressive psychotherapy evolved as a less intense version of psychoanalysis, more suitable for sicker patients.)

Psychoanalysis is intended to address long-standing unconscious conflicts and personality issues. Symptomatic relief is an expected by-product of this process but is not a short-term goal, so psychoanalysis is not suitable for patients with significant, acute Axis I disorders. Other factors limit its usefulness as well. The expense of the frequent sessions may be considerable and must usually be largely or entirely out of pocket. Also, patients with moderate to severe personality disorders, or with diatheses toward psychosis, are unlikely to tolerate the strong transference that emerges under the conditions of analysis. Therefore, most persons who undergo psychoanalysis are relatively healthy, with at most mild personality troubles or neurotic symptoms such as mild depression or anxiety. Most analytic patients also have high motivation for change and for exploration of their internal self.

BRIEF PSYCHODYNAMIC PSYCHOTHERAPY

Supportive-expressive psychotherapy can be and often is successfully used for a brief course, over perhaps 2 or 3 months. The following circumstances often apply:

- A discrete focal problem can be identified. The focal problem should be of recent onset or exacerbation and is often a response to a recent stressor. The "problem" may manifest as intrapsychic symptoms, interpersonal discord, or decline from baseline level of functioning in one or several life roles.
- The patient must be motivated to use psychotherapy.
- An explicit treatment "contract" is reached with the patient, wherein a set frequency and total duration of sessions is established, and the patient and therapist agree to work together on the focal problem. It is explicitly recognized that longer-term psychological issues may influence the focal problem and that areas that might benefit from longer-term therapy might be identified during this course of treatment. Such areas will merely be identified, however; the treatment will focus entirely on issues directly related to the focal problem.
- The therapist must decide in the assessment

or early treatment phase of the therapy how much to use interpretations (almost solely of the "here and now" variety) and harder-edged confrontations, and how much to rely on clarifications and guidance/recommendations. In other words, where on the supportive-expressive continuum will most of the work lie? The previously noted relative indications for supportive and expressive therapy apply here and are used to inform this decision.

BEHAVIORAL AND COGNITIVE PSYCHOTHERAPY

As mentioned briefly in Chapter 3, behavioral approaches to psychotherapy are rooted in learning theory. Reinforcement is used to promote desirable behaviors and to reduce undesirable ones. In essence, patients learn that they can endure feelings or circumstances that they previously thought unendurable and that they can get their emotional needs met without resorting to troublesome, undesired behavior. They learn this through a series of mental or action-oriented exercises, both in therapy sessions and in homework assignments between sessions.

Cognitive therapy helps patients alter dysfunctional patterns of thinking. It is rooted in cognitive psychology and, through psychoeducation and specific assignments (in sessions and between sessions), helps patients identify their cognitive distortions and replace them with more flexible thoughts that do not lead directly to the undesired symptoms.

As noted previously, in some ways cognitive therapy is a behavioral approach to thoughts rather than to external actions. Cognitive and behavioral approaches are often combined in clinical practice, hence the commonly used term *cognitive-behavioral therapy*. Therapists take an active approach in administering cognitive-behavioral therapy. They must offer considerable psychoeducation, reassurance, and positive expectations to maximize the likelihood that the patient will comply with the specific assignments and tasks. Thus, although the specific efficacy of these therapies results from particular techniques, their overall effectiveness depends on a positive treatment alliance as much as do psychodynamic psychotherapies and all other clinician-patient encounters.

Cognitive, behavioral, or cognitive-behavioral therapies are useful in a broad range of clinical circumstances:

- Specific phobias (the primary treatment)
- Most other anxiety disorders (may be a primary, co-primary, or adjunctive treatment)
- Anxiety symptoms as part of other psychiatric disorders
- Eating disorders
- Sexual dysfunctions
- Depressive syndromes
- Substance-use disorders
- Specific problematic behaviors (e.g., self-mutilation, aggressive outbursts) seen as part of a variety of organic mental syndromes, including developmental disorders (e.g., autism), mental retardation, dementias, or other secondary syndromes
- Specific problematic behaviors seen as part of a variety of idiopathic mental syndromes, including schizophrenia and personality disorders
- A variety of psychosomatic (or psychophysiological) disorders in which relaxation techniques or biofeedback may be useful, such as chronic headache or other pain syn-

dromes, hypertension, or irritable bowel syndrome

GROUP PSYCHOTHERAPY

A wide variety of groups are available to patients. All use the therapeutic leverage of the group process. That is, the sense of belonging to a group, gaining support from one's peers, and (in some groups) being confronted by one's peers can be enormously powerful in helping effect desired changes.

Groups may differ greatly along several dimensions, including:

- *Group leadership*. There are self-help groups and groups led by professionals of varied backgrounds, including (but not always limited to) psychotherapists.
- *Meeting times*. Group sessions may be 30 minutes or 8 hours long, although 1 to 1½ hours is probably the most common length. Most groups meet weekly, but many meet less often, and occasional groups meet more often.
- *Duration*. Groups may meet for a preestablished number of sessions or weeks, or may exist indefinitely.
- *Open or closed*. Some groups accept new members during their existence, but others are closed after forming. Similarly, many groups expect that some members will leave the group during the time of the group's existence, and others expect that the membership will remain stable.
- *Size*. Depending on a group's theoretical orientation and treatment goals, the number of members may vary greatly. Most profession-

ally led psychotherapy groups are of a size technically known as *small groups*, defined as being large enough to have true group dynamics (at least three or four members), but small enough so that each participant can maintain eye contact with all other participants (no more than about 12 members).

- *Setting and context.* Groups may serve outpatients; day or partial hospital patients; inpatients from psychiatric, rehabilitation, or other medical settings; or residents of a group home, nursing home, or other residential facility. A group may be a patient's sole treatment or may be used in combination with other groups (a *group program*) or other treatment modalities.

- *Homogeneous versus heterogeneous patient population.* Some groups select patients based on a common symptom, diagnosis, or demographic variable. Other groups, such as inpatient groups open to all patients on the unit, take all comers. Each of these approaches has its own leverages and disadvantages.

- *Theoretical orientations.* These may draw on any of the many perspectives discussed for individual psychotherapies. Most self-help groups are supportive in nature, although some may rely heavily on confrontation at times (e.g., Alcoholics Anonymous). Professionally led therapy groups may be based on supportive-expressive psychodynamic techniques, with awareness of the interpersonal dynamics within the group as a whole and the intrapsychic dynamics of each member. Other psychotherapy groups may use cognitive-behavioral approaches, essentially using group dynamics to support the psychoeducation and cognitive or behavioral assignments critical to these therapies. (Such groups are more likely to be diagnostically homogeneous, so that each member is working on similar assignments aimed at changing similar behaviors.) Activities-therapy groups may range from task oriented (e.g., arts and crafts) to more process and interpersonally oriented therapy groups utilizing music, art, or other modalities.

- *Goals.* As with individual psychotherapies, group therapy goals may range from highly specific (e.g., maintaining alcohol sobriety, decreasing the frequency of obsessions or compulsions) to broad (e.g., coping with chronic medical illness, fostering personal growth and maturation).

FAMILY THERAPY

Family therapies, of course, are theoretically based on family systems perspectives. In practice, conducting family therapy resembles conducting group therapy, particularly in the way in which the therapist must integrate consideration of each member as an individual with recognition of dynamics among members (including dyads, triangles, and the whole family). Unlike most group therapies, however, this particular group has a long and complex history that predates its contact with the therapist, and most interactions within this group take place outside of therapy sessions. In order to exert useful therapeutic leverage within the family, the therapist must understand the traditions and styles of each family and must eventually be seen by the family as (almost) one of them rather than purely as an outsider.

Families often enter family therapy with one

"identified patient" among them. That is, one particular family member is the most overtly symptomatic. The recognition of him or her as the "one with the problem" may be helpful or unhelpful for that person and the rest of the family. The identified patient may well be the most severely disordered family member, but the dynamics of family interactions may perpetuate or exacerbate the patient's symptoms. Addressing these interactions offers one route to reducing these symptoms and improving the overall course of illness.

As in the other psychotherapeutic modalities, family therapy may use any of a variety of techniques, including supportive, expressive, and cognitive-behavioral. However, the barriers among these perspectives may be even less rigid than in other modalities.

Family therapy does not have indications limited to specific diagnoses. Whatever the diagnosis of the identified patient, clinical assessment of the *family* leads to the recommendation for family work. Whether family therapy is a primary or adjunctive treatment depends on numerous clinical factors, including the patient's diagnosis, the amenability of the family to such therapy, and the relative amenability of the patient to individual or group work as alternatives. Family therapy is often crucial in working with children, adolescents, and geriatric patients, given both the nature of the disorders seen in these age groups and the developmental issues common at these ages, necessitating close ties to family members around illness-related symptoms or treatments. Research has also demonstrated the effectiveness of family therapy in other contexts. For example, using psychoeducational and supportive family therapy to reduce "expressed emotion" (openly expressed hostility or criticism) clearly reduces relapse in patients with schizophrenia or mood disorders.

One variant of family therapy is couples therapy. Often couples therapy is essentially straightforward, psychodynamically informed psychotherapy applied to a dyadic relationship. Sometimes couples therapy is more limited in focus and technique, such as behavioral approaches to sexual dysfunctions (sex therapy). As always, one should be flexible in tailoring the therapy to the patient's (or couple's) needs, rather than attempting to fit the patient into a rigid treatment strategy.

16
CHAPTER

Psychopharmacology and Electroconvulsive Therapy

Medications, electroconvulsive therapy (ECT), and other physical procedures (collectively known as "somatic therapies") are often used to treat psychiatric disorders. This chapter will begin with general guidelines to somatic treatments and then briefly consider the specific agents.

GENERAL GUIDELINES*

1. **Begin with the most accurate diagnosis or differential diagnosis possible.** Diagnosis will determine whether, when, what, and how drugs should be used.
2. **Pick and document the target symptoms.** The more specific you can be about which

---

*Adapted with permission from Guttmacher, LB: Concise Guide to Psychopharmacology and Electroconvulsive Therapy. American Psychiatric Press, Inc., Washington, DC, 1994, pp 1-8.

symptoms you hope to improve with treatment and how severe these symptoms are initially, the better you can monitor response to treatment and evaluate side effects.

3. **Obtain a detailed patient (and family) drug history.** "Detailed" includes information such as drug, dosage, duration, target symptoms, tolerability, response, and reason for discontinuation. If you obtain and use these data, you can save the patient considerable time or toxicity.

4. **Except in an emergency, don't alter a psychotropic regimen without completing steps 1 to 3.** *Corollary #1:* Don't start, stop, or change the dose of a drug just to "do something." (Or, as the wise saying goes, "Don't just do something—stand there!") *Corollary #2:* If your new-to-you patient is taking a psychotropic medication, stopping it before completing steps 1 to 3 will likely confuse you in assessing withdrawal effects versus symptoms of the underlying disorder.

5. **Changing one variable at a time maximizes your ability to definitively evaluate medication benefits and side effects.** Unfortunately from the perspective of pure science, and (often) fortunately from the perspective of timely patient care, we frequently institute a combination of psychopharmacological, psychotherapeutic, or social treatments. Just don't add to the mess by making any more medication changes at one time than necessary.

6. **Selection of drugs within a given class depends more on relative side effects than efficacy.** There is no reason to think that haloperidol is a more effective antipsychotic than molindone, or that amitriptyline is a more effective tricyclic antidepressant than desipramine. Yet differing relative side effect

profiles may strongly favor one over the other for a given patient. For instance, in an elderly depressed patient prone to delirium, desipramine (with its lower anticholinergic activity) is probably a better choice than amitriptyline.

7. **Selection of a particular drug class depends on diagnosis, target symptoms, and side effects and may also be reasonably affected by cost and personal preferences.** For example, for a patient with severe melancholic major depression, more data support the use of tricyclic or monoamine oxidase inhibitor (MAOI) antidepressants than the serotonin-specific reuptake inhibitors (SSRIs). For a mildly, nonmelancholically major depressed outpatient, however, efficacy studies do not offer a clear choice among tricyclics, SSRIs, bupropion, venlafaxine, or nefazodone. Side effect profiles, cost, and your own comfort with a particular agent will typically guide the choice of drug.

8. **In evaluating response and side effects, look at the forest as well as the trees.** The importance of the details (i.e., the quantity and quality of target symptoms) has already been noted. However, fluctuation of symptoms and behavior is the norm, not the exception. Unless the symptoms or behavior present an urgent need to act, try to judge the overall picture before adjusting dosage or abandoning a medication trial. In other words, ask both, "How does the patient look right at the moment?" and "How have the past few days (or weeks) gone, and how do they compare to the few days (or weeks) prior?"

9. **The rules of drug nonspecificity**
   a. *Drugs don't just treat one symptom or syndrome.* For example, antidepressants of

various classes may be used to treat depressive symptoms, panic attacks, social phobias, obsessions or compulsions, primary insomnia, enuresis, and other disorders.

b. *Drugs treat symptoms across diagnoses.* For example, antidepressants treat depressive symptoms in major depression, bipolar depression, depression secondary to Alzheimer's disease, and so forth. Antipsychotics treat psychotic symptoms due to schizophrenia, delusional disorder, mood disorders, delirium, dementias such as Alzheimer's disease, and so forth. Efficacy, toxicity, and dosage may vary greatly across diagnoses, however (hence the need for step 1).

c. *Drugs treat symptoms, not diagnoses.* For example, antipsychotics are far more effective with certain symptoms of schizophrenia than with others.

10. **Compliance is a major issue.** This statement is, of course, true for all clinical pharmacology but is especially relevant to psychopharmacology because:

a. *Side effects are common and often troubling to patients.*

b. *Impaired insight into the need for medications, or impaired ability to successfully stick to a medication schedule, are inherent in many psychiatric disorders.*

c. *Social stigma, including sometimes direct pressure from family or peers, may encourage patients to "work it out by themselves" or to avoid "mind-altering drugs."* Paying attention to all these factors, as they play out for each individual patient, is the key to improving compliance. Indeed, they are crucial to the quality of your relationship with your patient, which is the single strongest predictor of compliance.

    d. The positive effects of psychotropics are often delayed.

11. **Remember the almighty $.** Medications are expensive, particularly newer agents that do not have generic competition. Keep this in mind as you choose medications, and prescribe generics when possible. (Few clear data suggest differences in bioequivalence among various preparations, except for medications for children.)

12. **Don't polypharmacize.** There is never a good reason to prescribe more than one drug from the same class at the same time. There are lots of good reasons *not* to do so, all of which involve the concept of additive toxicity. (Please note that combining medications from *different* classes is another story, one that is often justified or even optimal.)

13. **Acute treatment ≠ maintenance treatment.** Most major psychiatric disorders tend to relapse or recur over time. Once your patient is better acutely, you must consciously decide—ideally in collegial discussion with the patient—whether to use maintenance medication to reduce the risks of recurrence. The choice of drug or dosage may differ depending on whether you are using the drug for acute or prophylactic treatment.

14. **Learn a few drugs from each class well.** The list of psychotropic medications is rather long, and the nonpsychiatric physician need not learn all of them. Indeed, since efficacy does not differ among drugs within a given class, even most psychiatrists need not gain great comfort with all of them. Become thoroughly familiar with a few representatives from each class. For example, one low-potency, one medium-potency, and one or two high-potency traditional neuroleptics

are plenty for most purposes. Admittedly, though, the number of new drugs that appear to be in their own classes structurally and clinically (e.g., risperidone, venlafaxine, nefazodone) is growing rapidly. This is probably good for our patients, if hard on our memories.

15. **Be skeptical of new products and trends (fads?) in prescribing practices.** It may take months or even a few years to really sort out a new drug's efficacy and toxicity and how it compares to previous agents. So, though you don't want to be the last doc on your block to prescribe a new drug, you shouldn't be the first to do so either.

16. **Remember the heterogeneity of group populations, a.k.a. "There are no rules."** Like most of medical practice, the empirical base of clinical psychopharmacology rests on studies of patient groups. Individual patients may vary, and your current patient may well be an outlier in terms of response, toxicity, dosage requirements, and so forth. This, of course, is what makes the practice of psychiatry and medicine maddening (in the nontechnical sense) or fun, depending on your viewpoint. (The latter perspective is highly recommended.)

SPECIFIC DRUG CLASSES

The following is intended as an orientation to the main types of drugs you will find used in psychiatric settings. It is neither an exhaustive list nor a substitute for a good reference text on psychopharmacology (such as the masterpiece cited on page 188).

Antipsychotics

Traditional Antipsychotics

Pharmacokinetics. Many antipsychotic, or neuroleptic, medications are available (Table 16–1). All are equally effective if given in equivalent doses, but potency varies widely. Relative potency is often denoted by comparison to 100 mg of chlorpromazine. All are lipophilic and hepatically metabolized. Half-lives vary among patients as well as among different agents, but they are in the range of at least 18 to 24 hours. (Translation: Once-daily dosing is usually sufficient and helps compliance.)

Availability. All are available in oral form, and some are also available for parenteral use. Intramuscular (IM) administration of low-potency neuroleptics such as chlorpromazine should be avoided when possible because of both the volume of vehicle needed and the possibility of uncomfortable local reactions. Two agents (fluphenazine and haloperidol) are available in esterified form (e.g., decanoate) for long-acting IM administration every 2 weeks (fluphenazine) or every 4 weeks (haloperidol), facilitating compliance.

Mechanism of Action. A real answer to this question would mean that we truly understood the pathophysiology of psychosis, which should earn us a Nobel prize at the least. But we do know that antipsychotic potency correlates roughly with the degree to which a drug blocks D_2-dopaminergic receptors. Unfortunately from the point of view of side effects, antipsychotics block most receptors under the sun, including muscarinic cholinergic, alpha$_1$-adrenergic, and histaminergic (especially H_1) receptors.

Indications. Indications include:

- Psychotic symptoms (as part of many disorders)
- Manic symptoms (as part of bipolar, schizoaffective, or secondary disorders)
- Acute impulse dyscontrol or affective instability or lability (e.g., as part of personality disorders under acute stressors, or in dementias or other secondary syndromes)
- Acute psychomotor agitation caused by the above or other syndromes
- Tics, choreiform movements, and some other adventitious movement disorders
- Nausea and vomiting (some agents, such as prochlorperazine [Compazine], are marketed specifically as antiemetics)
- Intractable and disabling hiccoughs (honestly!)

Time to Response. Sedative or antiagitation effects may begin within an hour after oral administration and considerably more rapidly after parenteral use. True antipsychotic effects may take several days or more to begin, and maximum antipsychotic benefit from a given dose may take 2 weeks or more. Given this, the common practice of using neuroleptics on a prn basis for psychosis is highly questionable (although prn use for agitation may be defensible in certain circumstances).

Side Effects. All these drugs have the same list of side effects but in different proportions. The general rule is that the high-potency antipsychotics have more extrapyramidal side effects (EPS), while the low-potency drugs have more of almost everything else. Side effects of antipsychotics may be obvious or subtle, may simulate the symptoms of the disorder you're trying to treat (e.g., akathisia may look like psychosis-

Table 16-1. SOME TRADITIONAL ANTIPSYCHOTICS

NAME (BRAND NAME)	CHEMICAL CLASS	APPROXIMATE CHLORPROMAZINE EQUIVALENTS (mg = 100 mg CPZ)	AVAILABLE PARENTERALLY?	COMMENTS
Chlorpromazine (Thorazine)	Aliphatic phenothiazine	100	Yes	IM injections require large amounts of fluid vehicle and may be painful
Mesoridazine (Serentil)	Piperidine phenothiazine	50	Yes	
Thioridazine (Mellaril)	Piperidine phenothiazine	95–100	No	Pigmentary retinopathy at > 800 mg/d
Fluphenazine (Prolixin)	Piperazine phenothiazine	2	Yes	Available as decanoate
Perphenazine (Trilafon)	Piperazine phenothiazine	8	Yes	

Trifluoperazine (Stelazine)	Piperazine phenothiazine	5	Yes	
Thiothixene (Navane)	Thioxanthene	5	Yes	
Loxapine (Loxitane)	Dibenzoxazepine	10–15	Yes	Chemically related to antidepressant amoxapine
Molindone (Moban)	Indolone	10	No	
Droperidol (Inapsine)	Butyrophenone	1–2	Yes	Parenteral only
Haloperidol (Haldol)	Butyrophenone	2–4	Yes	Available as decanoate
Pimozide (Orap)	Diphenylbutylpiperidine	1	No	

related psychomotor agitation), and are contributors to medication noncompliance. They include:

- EPS. These come in both acute and delayed varieties. The acute forms include *dystonias* (sustained muscle contractions that may be painful); *akathisia* (motor restlessness, often manifested as pacing, rocking, or other symmetric/rhythmic motions); and *parkinsonism* (which, like the manifestations of idiopathic Parkinson's disease, includes bradykinesia, rigidity, festinating gait, and drooling). The delayed forms of EPS usually occur after months or years of exposure, and in some cases may not be reversible even if the medication is discontinued. Most common is *tardive dyskinesia*, but *tardive dystonia* and *tardive akathisia* have also been described.
- Neuroleptic malignant syndrome (NMS). Closely related to the standard EPS, this potentially life-threatening syndrome is thought to be an idiosyncratic drug reaction. See Chapter 18 for further details.
- Anticholinergic effects. The usual list, including dry mouth, constipation, blurry vision, urinary retention, tachycardia, potential to precipitate an episode of narrow angle glaucoma, and delirium. (Remember "dry as a bone, red as a beet, blind as a bat, mad as a hatter"?)
- Orthostatic hypotension (probably related to alpha$_1$-adrenergic blockade).
- Sedation.
- Skin: allergic rashes (as may be seen with many drugs); photosensitivity, such that patients should take care to use extra ultraviolet protection if exposed to sunlight.
- Ocular pigmentation (including pigmentary retinopathy, which is seen with thioridazine at doses above 800 mg/day).
- Galactorrhea (because dopamine inhibits

prolactin release from the pituitary, and neuroleptics block dopamine).

- Weight gain (a longer-term side effect).
- Nonspecific electrocardiogram (ECG) changes, including ST-segment and T-wave alterations, which are rarely of any clinical significance. In overdosage, widening of PR or QT intervals, or other arrhythmias, may be seen with low-potency antipsychotics.
- Hepatic toxicity. Cholestatic jaundice is the classic picture described with low-potency agents, but all neuroleptics may also cause elevation of hepatocellular enzymes, usually without clinical significance beyond the need for monitoring.
- Seizures. Lowering of seizure threshold is described for nearly all psychotropics (except for the anticonvulsants, of course), including the neuroleptics.
- Agranulocytosis. Rare, and probably limited to the older low-potency phenothiazines.
- Sexual dysfunctions, including retrograde ejaculation (particularly with the older, lower-potency drugs).

Newer Antipsychotics

Two newer antipsychotic agents, clozapine and risperidone, have been introduced to the U.S. market (as usual, later than in other countries). Both have side effect profiles similar to those of traditional antipsychotics, with the substantial exception that EPS are rare or nonexistent at conventional dosing. (This probably also means that the long-term risk of tardive dyskinesia is extraordinarily low.) Clozapine has been demonstrated to reduce psychotic symptoms in schizophrenic patients previously resistant to several adequate trials of traditional neuroleptics. However, it produces potentially life-threatening agranulocytosis often enough that weekly monitoring of the complete blood count (CBC) is required for as long as the patient takes the drug. Risperidone does not have this disadvantage. Whether it is as effective as clozapine in treatment-refractory patients is not yet clear. Also, higher doses of risperidone appear quite capable of producing EPS, removing some of its advantage over traditional neuroleptics.

By the time you read this, several additional "atypical" antipsychotics will have reached the U.S. market. Each shows promise in clinical trials to date. With the increasing number of antipsychotic alternatives, clinicians will need to hope for more comparative empiric studies to guide their choice of drugs for specific patient circumstances.

Antidepressants

General Considerations

The number and classes of antidepressant drugs have grown rapidly in the last 10 years. We'll consider some specific agents in a moment (or however long it takes you to finish reading this section).

Pharmacokinetics. All antidepressant drugs are lipophilic, and metabolism depends to a greater or lesser extent on hepatic oxidation, conjugation, and excretion. Half-lives vary, but for many drugs, they are long enough to allow once-daily (tricyclics, fluoxetine) or bid dosing. More frequent dosing is required only if peak-level side effects are troublesome. Bupropion does typically require tid dosing, as described later.

Availability. For all practical purposes in the U.S., none of these drugs are used (or available) in parenteral form. A working gastrointestinal tract and the willingness to swallow (or an enteral tube) are required.

Mechanism of Action. This remains unclear, reflecting our fundamental ignorance of the neurobiologic mechanisms of depression. All facilitate monoamine activity, particularly that of norepinephine or serotonin, doing so by reuptake blockade (tricyclics, SSRIs, venlafaxine), MAO inhibition (MAOIs), or several less clear mechanisms (bupropion, trazodone, nefazodone). Interestingly, direct agonists or stimulants that promote release of endogenous catecholamines tend to be unhelpful as primary antidepressant treatments (see Psychostimulants, later in this chapter).

Indications. Psychiatric indications for antidepressants include:

- Major depressive syndrome as part of major depressive, bipolar, or schizoaffective disorders, secondary mood disorders, dementia, or just about anything else except delirium (not that major depressive syndrome isn't seen in delirium—you just don't want to worsen the delirium by adding another drug that's active on the central nervous system [CNS]). Note that subtypes of depression (e.g., psychotic depression, melancholia), may have specific implications for the choice of an antidepressant or the need for combination therapy with other agents.
- Other, less severe depressive syndromes, such as dysthymic disorder or secondary mood disorders, that do not meet criteria for major depressive syndrome. (Both efficacy and the empirical support for these indications are lower than for major depression.)
- Panic disorder (best demonstrated: tricyclics, MAOIs, SSRIs)

- The "positive" symptoms of post-traumatic stress disorder (PSTD; best demonstrated: tricyclics, MAOIs)
- Obsessive-compulsive disorder (OCD— SSRIs, clomipramine)
- Social phobia (MAOIs)
- Acute cocaine craving (tricyclics)
- Eating disorders
- Attention deficit/hyperactivity disorder (probably; i.e., some evidence supports this indication)

Other conditions that may benefit from antidepressants include:

- Prophylaxis of chronic headaches of muscle tension or (some) of migraine-spectrum origin (tricyclics, probably SSRIs)
- Neuropathic pain syndromes (tricyclics; role of newer agents not clear)
- Insomnia, as a primary treatment in transient psychophysiological insomnia and an adjunctive treatment in other insomnias (any sedating antidepressant, e.g., trazodone, amitriptyline, doxepin)
- Enuresis (the most powerfully anticholinergic tricyclics, e.g., amitriptyline, doxepin)

Time to Response. Despite the claims of occasional drug advertisements, no class of antidepressants clearly works any faster than the others. For all, initial improvement may take at least 10 to 14 days (although some patients appear to improve more quickly), and maximum benefit may take 4 to 6 weeks or more.

Side Effects. Side effects vary by drug class and will be discussed in the sections below.

Choosing Which Drug to Use. Efficacy in outpatients with nonpsychotic, nonmelancholic major depression is probably about the same for all classes, although MAOIs *may* be more effective than others. However, an individual patient may respond poorly to one class and well to another, so in practice you must undertake a series of empirical trials to figure out what works for a given patient. Past response to antidepressants and (maybe) response of family members may be used to guide current treatment.

Major depression with psychotic features requires combination treatment with an antidepressant and an antipsychotic (or ECT). Best studied are tricyclics or MAOIs and traditional neuroleptics. There are few or no data regarding newer antidepressant classes in psychotic depression.

For patients with severe major depression, especially psychiatric inpatients or those with melancholia, again the best studied treatments are tricyclics, MAOIs, and ECT. There are fewer or no data regarding newer antidepressant classes, although preliminary evidence supports a role for venlafaxine.

Patients with depression who fail to obtain remission with single antidepressant agents may benefit from adding a second antidepressant ("combination strategies") or by adding a drug that by itself is a poor antidepressant ("augmentation," such as with lithium, triiodothyronine, or psychostimulants). There is growing empirical support for several augmentation strategies, but data are more limited regarding combination approaches. Of course, with the rapidly expanding arsenal of antidepressant drugs and classes, the permutations of combinations are increasing too. Pending clearer empirically supported directions, these strategies should mostly be reserved for use by psychiatrists with selected treatment-refractory patients.

Tricyclics

Although they're called "tricyclics" in common usage, some of these drugs don't have three rings (e.g., the tetracyclic maprotiline).

Side Effects. The side effect profile for tricyclics is long and appears forbidding, but most patients tolerate them fairly well. Side effects include:

- Anticholinergic effects, such as constipation, dry mouth, urine retention, blurry vision, precipitation of acute-angle glaucoma (note that there is *no* contraindication in the far more common open-angle glaucoma), sinus tachycardia, delirium.
- Orthostatic hypotension.
- Sedation.
- Cardiac conduction effects. Tricyclics are essentially class Ia antiarrhythmics. They are absolutely contraindicated in patients with bifascicular blocks (e.g., left bundle-branch block [LBBB] plus first-degree atrioventricular [AV] block), and must be used with caution in patients with more worrisome monofascicular blocks (e.g., LBBB, or second-degree AV block). Older patients and those with known heart disease should have baseline ECGs before initiating tricyclic therapy, and the ECGs should be monitored during treatment, paying special attention to PR, QRS, and QT intervals.
- Potential lethality in overdose, with severe cardiac conduction abnormalities, other arrhythmias, seizures, or cardiovascular collapse.
- Sympathomimetic effects. Often minimal, but prominent in some patients, these may include diaphoresis, postural tremor, and anxiety.
- Weight gain over the longer term.

- Sexual dysfunctions, including anorgasmia.
- Lowering of seizure threshold.

Choosing the Right Dosage. It becomes apparent that monitoring blood levels is crucial to proper dosing of tricyclics if we put together three facts:

1. The rate of tricyclic metabolism varies enormously among patients.
2. Efficacy depends on blood level.
3. Although side effects depend on dose and level, it is difficult to correlate them with specific blood levels in a population.

Desipramine levels should be greater than 125 ng/mL, while nortriptyline has a therapeutic window between 50 and 150 ng/mL. Imipramine should result in a combined imipramine/desipramine level of greater than 225 ng/mL. Data on therapeutic levels are few for other tricyclics, so don't waste a blood test on them unless you're trying to figure out if the patient took an overdose or is taking the drug at all.

Choosing Which Drug to Use. See Table 16–2 for a list of generic and brand names. Do not memorize this list, because in almost all cases it makes sense to use nortriptyline, desipramine, or imipramine if you're going to use a tricyclic at all. (All tricyclics have the same efficacy if used in equivalent doses, so you might as well become comfortable using a couple of them and forget about the rest.) Although desipramine and nortriptyline share the same side effect profile as the other tricyclics, they have *less* of these side effects than most others. For most patients this is a good thing. (For a few it is not; if you're using a tricyclic specifically as a hypnotic or an anticholinergic, such as for enuresis, amitriptyline or doxepin would be better choices.) Also, data on blood levels and treatment response are

Table 16-2. SOME "TRI"CYCLIC ANTIDEPRESSANTS

NAME (BRAND NAME)	CHEMICAL CLASS	TYPICAL DOSAGE RANGE*	COMMENTS
Nortriptyline (Pamelor, Aventyl)	Secondary amine tricyclic	50–150 mg/d	Therapeutic plasma level 50–150 ng/mL
Desipramine (Norpramin, Pertofrane)	Secondary amine tricyclic	150–300 mg/d	Therapeutic plasma level >125 ng/mL
Protriptyline (Vivactyl)	Secondary amine tricyclic	10–40 mg/d	Highly activating (may be a limiting side effect)
Imipramine (Tofranil)	Tertiary amine tricyclic	150–300 mg/d	Therapeutic plasma level >225 ng/mL (combined imipramine and desipramine level)

Amitriptyline (Elavil)	Tertiary amine tricyclic	150–300 mg/d	Therapeutic plasma level unclear; although many labs will report combined amitriptyline and nortriptyline level
Doxepin (Sinequan)	Tertiary amine tricyclic	150–300 mg/d	
Clomipramine (Anafranil)	Tertiary amine tricyclic	150–300 mg/d	Structurally a tricyclic, has tricyclic side effects, but is a serotonin-specific reuptake inhibitor (e.g., used to treat obsessive-compulsive disorder)
Maprotiline (Ludiomil)	Tetracyclic	50–200 mg/d	
Amoxapine (Asendin)	Dibenzoxazepine (heterocyclic)	150–300 mg/d	Chemically related to the antipsychotic loxapine; may have neuroleptic-like side effects including potential for tardive dyskinesia

* But REMEMBER enormous variability among patients!

clearer for desipramine, nortriptyline, and imipramine than for other tricyclics; as mentioned above, use of blood levels is often quite helpful. Imipramine and amitriptyline are metabolized to desipramine and nortriptyline, respectively, so why not eliminate the middleman?

If cost is a more important issue than side effects, imipramine may be the best choice. Although available generically, nortriptyline is fairly expensive, and even desipramine is not as cheap as some other tricyclics (especially imipramine and amitriptyline); financial concerns are perhaps the best reason *not* to choose nortriptyline or desipramine with certain patients.

SSRIs

Currently available SSRIs are fluoxetine (Prozac), sertraline (Zoloft), paroxetine (Paxil), and fluvoxamine (Luvox). Luvox has received FDA approval to be marketed for the treatment of OCD, but all are effective in treating depression, OCD, and possibly other conditions as described previously. Fluoxetine's metabolites have half-lives measured in weeks, which may pose a problem with drug interactions when switching to different agents.

Clomipramine is a serotonin-reuptake blocker and hence is effective in OCD as well as depression. However, in structure and side effect profile it is a tricyclic (it is actually chlorinated imipramine), and so it is not usually considered an SSRI.

The SSRIs are relatively easy to administer, based on standard doses or dosing ranges. Blood levels are not clinically useful at this time.

Side Effects. The side effect profile of SSRIs is in most respects more benign than that of tricyclics, and most patients tolerate them quite well. Clinical experience suggests that older patients, or those with neurological disease, may be more susceptible to CNS side effects. The profile includes:

- Anorexia and (usually limited) weight loss (note that patients who have anorexia as part of their depression and who respond to the SSRI will indeed have improved appetite).
- Insomnia (but ditto regarding improvement in sleep when the patient improves).
- Nausea, and less often, vomiting.
- Headache.
- Sexual dysfunctions, including anorgasmia, ejaculatory delay, and decreased libido.
- CNS effects, including anxiety, increased arousal or jitteriness, akathisia or similar states of increased psychomotor activity, delirium (this last usually in patients with preexisting brain disease).
- Inhibition of certain cytochrome P450 isozymes, leading to clinically meaningful rises in blood levels of other drugs metabolized by this system. This effect may be less severe with sertraline and fluvoxamine.

Bupropion

Bupropion (Wellbutrin) is probably as good a choice as an SSRI for first-line treatment of uncomplicated outpatient major depression. Its most significant practical liability is the need for multiple daily dosing. Note also that bupropion is probably the only important antidepressant on the market that does *not* effectively treat panic disorder.

Because of the risk of seizures, dosing needs to be as follows: no more than 150 mg/single dose, and no more than 450 mg/day total. Since the target dose is usually 300 to 450 mg/day, bid or tid dosing is required. Used in this manner, bupropion probably poses no greater risk of seizures than other antidepressants for patients without premorbid conditions that put them at higher seizure risk. For unclear reasons, patients with eating disorders have a greater incidence of seizures with bupropion.

Side Effects. Bupropion is generally well tolerated, but potential side effects in addition to seizures include:

- Stimulant-like effects, including psychomotor agitation, insomnia, anxiety, tremor
- Nausea
- Headaches

MAOIs

Availability. Only two MAOIs currently marketed in the U.S. are effective antidepressants: phenelzine (Nardil) and tranylcypromine (Parnate). These are both mixed inhibitors; that is, they inhibit both MAO-A and MAO-B. MAO-B–selective inhibitors such as selegiline (Eldepryl) appear to be ineffective as antidepressants. Newer MAOIs, including reversible MAO-A inhibitors, may reach the U.S. market in the foreseeable future.

Indications. MAOIs *may* be more effective than other antidepressant medications in major depression and certain anxiety disorders such as panic disorder or social phobia. Some studies suggest that MAOIs are preferentially effective in major depression with prominent anxiety, reversed neurovegetative signs (e.g., hypersomnia, hyperphagia, weight gain), or sensitivity to interpersonal rejection.

Like tricyclics, MAOIs have a longer and better track record than newer agents in patients with melancholia or psychotic depression, including severely depressed inpatients.

Side Effects. The only reason MAOIs are not prescribed more often is the need for a tyramine-free diet. In other words, patients have to be capable and willing to follow the diet, and not suicidal enough to intentionally eat the wrong foods. Tyramine is an amino acid found in certain foods. When these foods are ingested, the tyramine is normally metabolized in the gut by MAO-A. If MAO-A is inhibited by an MAOI drug, the tyramine is absorbed and then (probably with help from some other vasoactive amines) promotes rapid release of endogenous catecholamines, leading to a hypertensive crisis. Foods that must be avoided include cheeses (except cottage and cream cheese); fermented or cured meats (including bologna, salami, pepperoni); dried or cured fish; fava beans; figs; and many wines and beers (although most persons with depression needing MAOI treatment shouldn't be drinking alcohol anyway).

The clinical presentation of a hypertensive crisis is what you would expect from sympathomimetic hyperactivity: malignant hypertension (with attendant manifestations including headache, nausea/vomiting, angina, or stroke), tachycardia, diaphoresis, fever, and cardiac arrhythmias.

Sympathomimetic drugs can obviously contribute to an MAOI crisis and must be avoided. Caffeine (e.g., coffee, chocolate) probably should be taken in moderation. Patients need to be warned about over-the-counter medications, including diet pills (stimulants) and cold/cough preparations that contain decongestants. In addition to prescription sympathomimetics, most opioids need to be avoided, particularly meperidine (Demerol), although morphine has been used safely when necessary.

As well, a washout period is advised when switching to or from MAOIs and most other antidepressant classes.

If the diet is followed, MAOIs are generally well tolerated. Additional side effects include:

- Stimulant-like effects, such as insomnia, anxiety, tremor, diaphoresis, myoclonic jerks (all more common with tranylcypromine than phenelzine)
- Orthostatic hypotension
- Sexual dysfunctions (impotence, anorgasmia)
- Weight gain
- Anticholinergic effects (although much less so than with tricyclics)
- Hepatitis (more so with phenelzine)

Trazodone and Nefazodone

Trazodone (Desyrel) was one of the first newer antidepressants to be marketed. Unfortunately, anecdotal experience has led many clinicians to believe that it is less effective than other antidepressants, especially for moderate to severe major depression. It is quite sedating, which leads to its most common current usage as a hypnotic, often as an adjunct to stimulating antidepressants such as SSRIs and MAOIs. Other side effects include orthostatic hypotension and (rare but severe) priapism.

Nefazodone (Serzone) is an analogue of trazodone but appears to be as effective as other antidepressants in treating all forms of major depression. It has only relatively recently come to market, but it appears to be well tolerated. Certainly it is less sedating than trazodone, and it does not cause orthostatic hypotension in most patients.

Venlafaxine

Venlafaxine (Effexor) is a newer antidepressant with demonstrated effectiveness in a range of major depression severities. The side effect profile largely mimics that of the SSRIs, and it also may produce sustained *increases* in systemic blood pressure.

Psychostimulants

The most commonly used drugs in this class are methylphenidate (Ritalin), dextroamphetamine (Dexedrine), and pemoline (Cylert). All facilitate the transmission of endogenous catecholamines.

Indications. Indications include:

- Attention deficit/hyperactivity disorder (leading to improvement in attention, hyperactivity, and cognitive performance). These are all well documented effects, notwithstanding the claims of a few vocal persons or groups in the lay press.
- Depressive symptoms. Efficacy as a primary treatment in major depression is probably poor, but stimulants may be useful adjuncts when added to traditional antidepressants. They also may be helpful in older, medically ill patients without full-fledged major depressive syndromes, but with prominent anergia, amotivation, and psychomotor slowing.
- Narcolepsy.

Side Effects. Side effects are as you would predict for sympathomimetics (as for MAOIs). They also may produce anorexia, other gastrointestinal symptoms, or weight loss.

Mood Stabilizers (Thymoleptics)

General Considerations

Drugs with demonstrated thymoleptic efficacy include lithium, carbamazepine (Tegretol), and valproic acid (Depakene, Depakote). Other agents have been speculated to have such efficacy (e.g., calcium channel blockers), but data to support their use are few at this time.

Mechanism of Action. Even less is known about the mechanism of action for these drugs than for antidepressants. Delineation of a common mechanism, if there is one, is made complex by the disparity between lithium, a cation, and two lipophilic anticonvulsants. As a cation that may compete or substitute at ion channels or receptor sites, lithium potentially affects a wide range of neurobiologic activity, but the most salient effects are not known. The efficacy of anticonvulsant agents in bipolar disorder has led to "kindling" theories of mood disorders (i.e., that repeated activation of involved neural pathways leads to easier reactivation, or "kindling"), analogous to models of seizure disorders.

Indications. Data regarding efficacy in bipolar disorder for anticonvulsants are more recent, and therefore fewer, but clearly support their comparability to lithium and also suggest the usefulness of combining lithium and an anticonvulsant in treatment-refractory cases. Data regarding thymoleptic use in other psychiatric syndromes are mostly anecdotal or scarce with a few exceptions for lithium and carbamazepine.

Indications for mood stabilizers include:

- Bipolar disorder: acute treatment of manic or mixed episodes; prophylaxis of manic and depressive episodes; "coverage" to prevent antidepressant-induced manic swings during treatment of depressive episodes; augmentation of antidepressants for treatment of acute depression

- Bipolar II disorder and cyclothymic disorder: similar indications to those in bipolar I disorder, but data are fewer and efficacy may be less
- Unipolar major depression: augmentation of antidepressants for acute treatment (lithium); prophylaxis of recurrent episodes (lithium)
- Schizoaffective disorder: treatment of mood symptoms analogous to indications in bipolar disorder; also adjunctive treatment (along with antipsychotics) for psychotic symptoms
- Schizophrenia: adjunctive treatment (along with antipsychotics) for psychotic symptoms (lithium); probably works best in patients with some mood symptoms
- Long-term treatment of aggressivity, other impulse dyscontrol, or affective dysregulation in a variety of disorders, including mental retardation, developmental disorders, dementias, other secondary disorders (e.g., secondary personality change), conduct disorders, and personality disorders (all thymoleptics have been used, in most cases with limited anecdotal data or open trials to support their use)

Time to Response. In most uses (e.g., in acute mania), mood stabilizers act relatively slowly, and must be evaluated over at least 10 to 14 days to assess acute effects, hence the common practice of using neuroleptics or other agents initially for more rapid effects. To assess their effectiveness in more chronic states (e.g., chronic episodic aggressivity) or as prophylaxis, one must evaluate over several weeks or even months.

Lithium

Unlike most psychotropics, lithium is a cation, and therefore is hydrophilic and renally excreted. Lithium's half-life (approximately 24 hours in patients with normal renal function) would theoretically allow once-a-day dosing. In practice, peak-level side effects make bid dosing better tolerated. Only a few patients have enough trouble with peak side effects to necessitate tid or qid dosing; the common use of such dosing schedules seems hard to defend (unless you're in favor of encouraging poor medication compliance).

Choosing the Right Dosage. Lithium has a low therapeutic index; that is, toxicity occurs at levels not very much higher than therapeutic levels, so one must be aware of fluctuations in lithium blood level. Conditions or drugs that may raise the lithium level include dehydration (e.g., excessive fluid losses on a hot day), other hypovolemic states, diuretics (especially those, such as thiazides, that act on the distal tubule), and nonsteroidal anti-inflammatory agents.

Published guides to therapeutic lithium levels, which usually claim a therapeutic range of 0.6 to 1.2, mEq/L are just that: guides. Individuals vary enormously in their ability to tolerate various levels and in what levels are required for efficacy. Even in the same patient, required levels depend on the therapeutic goal, such as:

- Higher levels (1.0 mEq/L and up) for acute mania
- Moderate levels (0.6–0.8 mEq/L) for prophylaxis (though some patients may require higher levels for maintenance)
- Low-moderate levels (0.5 mEq/L or so) for augmentation in unipolar depression

One specific opinion will be offered here: Many patients with acute mania are *under*treated. Response to lithium will be faster and more complete if the dose is pushed as high as the patient can tolerate, even if this results in a level that is "too high" on paper (not uncommonly 1.4 mEq/L or more for the acute manic phase).

Side Effects. The following list shows potential side effects of lithium, beginning with the more common side effects that may be seen at therapeutic levels and moving to the toxicities seen at supratherapeutic levels, including overdoses:

- Gastrointestinal: nausea, diarrhea, anorexia, vomiting
- Endocrinologic: hypothyroidism, goiter
- Cardiac: nonspecific T-wave changes, sinus arrhythmias
- Dermatologic: exacerbations of acne, psoriasis, or other chronic conditions; rashes of other types (e.g., maculopapular rash, folliculitis, [rare] exfoliative dermatitis)
- Renal: nephrogenic diabetes insipidus, proteinuria (which can rarely reach nephrotic syndrome levels), elevated serum creatinine/renal failure (rare except at toxic lithium levels)
- Hematologic: benign leukocytosis
- Neurological: tremor (typically position-holding), cognitive or psychomotor slowing, neuromuscular irritability, dysarthria, ataxia, delirium, seizures (these latter symptoms all being signs of worrisome toxicity)

From this list, the things to watch over the longer haul include thyroid and renal dysfunction.

Patients may develop tolerance to some of the above side effects, such as nausea. Reducing dosage when possible, or using divided doses to reduce peak level effects, is also helpful. If the effectiveness of the lithium warrants its continued use, some side effects may be treated with additional medications: thiazides or amiloride for nephrogenic diabetes insipidus (but lower the lithium dose to maintain the same blood level), beta blockers for tremor, or thyroid replacement for hypothyroidism.

For young and otherwise healthy patients, a screening and annual or biannual urinalysis plus serum creatinine and thyroid-stimulating hormone (TSH) levels are sufficient for the laboratory workup and monitoring, in addition to lithium levels. Despite its side effects and concerns about blood levels, lithium remains a useful and effective drug that is well tolerated by many patients.

Carbamazepine

Indications. Carbamazepine may be effective in patients for whom lithium is ineffective or intolerable. It is often well tolerated by patients, in particular having fewer CNS side effects at commonly used blood levels.

Choosing the Right Dosage. The therapeutic range of carbamazepine blood levels was established for use in epilepsy. It may be used as a rough guide for psychiatric use, but some patients will show benefit at low levels (especially when used in combination with lithium or other drugs), and others will tolerate and get additional benefit from high levels.

Side Effects. Side effects may include:

- Neurological: sedation, ataxia, dysarthria, delirium
- Hematologic: benign dyscrasias (particularly leukopenia), which should not be confused with the feared-but-fortunately-rare occurrence of idiosyncratic severe cell line depletions including aplastic anemia
- Gastrointestinal: nausea, dyspepsia

- Cardiac: conduction system disturbances (carbamazepine is structurally related to the tricyclic antidepressants)
- Dermatologic: rashes, from benign to exfoliative syndromes
- Hepatic: hepatitis

Valproic Acid

Indications. Valproate has similar psychiatric indications as carbamazepine, albeit usually with fewer data supporting its use. Some recent data suggest that it may work more rapidly than lithium in acute mania; it's unclear what to make of this yet, but the pharmaceutical companies' sales representatives must be thrilled.

Side Effects. It is usually well tolerated. The side effect profile is similar to that of carbamazepine, but aplastic anemia does not appear to be a risk. Hepatic toxicity may be a particular problem in children.

As with carbamazepine, blood levels are only a very rough guide to the benefit/side effects ratio for a given patient.

Anxiolytics

Benzodiazepines

Benzodiazepines have become the most popular of all the anxiolytics—and indeed among the most prescribed medications of any kind—because of their efficacy and relatively benign side effect profile, including (relative) safety in overdose.

Mechanism of Action. Benzodiazepines appear to act as agonists at sites in the benzodiazepine–gamma-aminobutyric acid (GABA) receptor complex, augmenting the activity of the inhibitory neurotransmitter GABA.

Indications. Indications for benzodiazepines include:

- Primary treatment for anxiety symptoms in panic disorder, generalized anxiety disorder, and situation-specific anxiety (including that associated with acute medical illnesses, procedures, and hospitalizations)
- Adjunctive treatment for anxiety symptoms in a wide range of other conditions, perhaps most notably in major depression
- Insomnia, either as primary treatment (e.g., transient psychophysiological insomnia) or as an adjunct during initial treatment of mood, psychotic, and other disorders (although only a few benzodiazepines are specifically marketed as hypnotics, any might be used; choice depends on pharmacokinetic profile and local practice patterns)
- Adjunctive treatment of psychomotor agitation in acute psychotic or manic states (indeed, benzodiazepine use may allow effective acute patient management with less overall neuroleptic exposure)
- Neuroleptic-induced akathisia, although other agents (e.g., beta-adrenergic blockers) are usually preferable
- Primary treatment of alcohol, barbiturate, or benzodiazepine withdrawal (there is cross-tolerance among benzodiazepines, barbiturates, and alcohol, so that administering any of these will lessen withdrawal symptoms from the others)
- Other uses that exploit properties such as muscle relaxation (e.g., diazepam for muscle spasms after acute back injury) and sedative/hypnotic/amnestic effects (e.g., midazolam for brief medical procedures)

Side Effects. Side effects include:

- Neurological: sedation, dysarthria, ataxia (beware of increased risk of falls!), delirium, hallucinosis.
- Psychiatric: cognitive slowing, amnesia, or global impairment (i.e., delirium); disinhibition (increased impulsivity or aggressivity, akin to what may be seen in ethanol intoxication).
- Dependency: Patients taking sufficient doses for long enough will develop physiological dependency; withdrawal symptoms resemble those of alcohol or barbiturate withdrawal. Patients also may become psychologically dependent on benzodiazepines; they become accustomed to (or enjoy) the feelings the drugs induce, and may seek higher doses or resist attempts to decrease or stop drug intake.

There are remarkably few other side effects. In particular, effects on pulse, blood pressure, cardiac output, and respiratory function are minimal in all but severe overdoses and rapid intravenous (IV) administrations.

Choosing Which Drug to Use. There are numerous benzodiazepines, as listed in Table 16–3. All are probably equally effective at equivalent doses, despite previous suggestions of preferential effects of alprazolam (Xanax) in panic disorder. All have common therapeutic properties as anxiolytics, hypnotics, and muscle relaxants. They vary in pharmacokinetics including half-life and presence of active metabolites (which may prolong the effective half-life even more).

Lorazepam is a high-potency benzodiazepine. Available in oral and parenteral forms, it is the only benzodiazepine that is consistently well absorbed IM. It is one of the few that is metabolized by direct conjugation, not requiring hepatic

Table 16-3. SOME BENZODIAZEPINES

NAME (BRAND NAME)	Mg POTENCY EQUIVALENCE (TO DIAZEPAM 5 mg)	ELIMINATION HALF-LIFE (HOURS) (INCLUDING ACTIVE METABOLITES)	ACTIVE METABOLITES?	COMMENTS
Diazepam (Valium)	5	30–200	Yes	
Chlordiazepoxide (Librium)	10	30–200	Yes	
Flurazepam (Dalmane)	30	50–200	Yes	

Temazepam (Restoril)	15	10–20	Yes	
Oxazepam (Serax)	15	5–20	No	
Clorazepate (Tranxene)	7.5	30–200	Yes	
Lorazepam (Ativan)	1	10–20	No	Well absorbed IM
Alprazolam (Xanax)	0.5	6–15	Yes	
Triazolam (Halcion)	0.125	1.5–3	Yes	
Clonazepam (Klonopin)	0.25	30	Yes	
Midazolam (Versed)	1(?)	1–12	No	For parenteral use only

oxidation, and does not have active metabolites. Given all these facts, you should make it one of the benzodiazepines you become experienced and comfortable prescribing.

Other Drugs

The following is an arbitrary, nonexhaustive, brief reference to other psychotropic agents and to nonpsychotropics that may have special or prominent uses in psychiatry.

Amantadine

This is both an antiviral agent (e.g., for influenza) and a treatment for Parkinson's disease. It promotes dopaminergic activity, probably by affecting reuptake mechanisms. It is used to treat neuroleptic-induced parkinsonism. Side effects are typically few and mild.

Anticholinergics

These drugs, such as benztropine (Cogentin) and trihexyphenidyl (Artane), block muscarinic receptors both centrally and peripherally. The central actions are responsible for their efficacy in neuroleptic-induced extrapyramidal side effects. They are especially useful for dystonia (parenterally for acute, severe dystonic reactions) and parkinsonism, and may be less effective in akathisia. Central actions may also lead to side effects including sedation, cognitive slowing, or frank delirium (quite common in older patients and those with premorbid brain disease). Peripheral cholinergic blockade causes side effects including dry mouth, constipation, urinary retention, tachycardia, blurry vision, and risk of precipitating acute-angle glaucoma. The potential for side effects, balanced against the discomfort of neuroleptic side effects (which may lead to noncompliance), has led to healthy debate about the merits of using anticholinergics prophylactically in patients begun on antipsychotics.

Beta-adrenergic Blockers

These drugs have two main psychiatric uses. The first is to treat neuroleptic-induced akathisia. The second is to treat the peripheral manifestations of situational anxiety in circumstances where benzodiazepines might be contraindicated (e.g., stage fright in a musician). Most reports on these uses have used propanolol, but it appears that other beta blockers, including those that do not cross the blood-brain barrier (e.g., atenolol) also work.

Buspirone

Buspirone (BuSpar) is a unique anxiolytic: It is not sedating, and physiological dependency does not develop. It does not have acute effects on anxiety, but may be effective for longer-term management of generalized anxiety disorder. Whether it is as effective as benzodiazepines is not clear. Patients experienced with the benzodiazepines often do not like BuSpar, perhaps partly because they are accustomed to the acute sense of a drug effect with each dose. BuSpar has also been used for other anxiety, depressive, and secondary mental disorders, although few data support these indications at this time.

Clonidine

Clonidine decreases central noradrenergic activity. Its most common use is as an antihypertensive. Significant data support its use in suppressing the symptoms of opioid withdrawal. It may have a role in the treatment of other withdrawal states (e.g., nicotine, alcohol), and in other psychiatric disorders with manifestations related to adrenergically mediated activity (e.g., anxiety disorders such as PSTD or panic disorder).

Diphenhydramine

Diphenhydramine (Benadryl), and other antihistamines as well, have been used as anxiolytics, hypnotics, and drugs to treat extrapyramidal side effects of neuroleptics. Try not to make these mistakes in your own practice. They are lousy anxiolytics. They offer no advantages over the anticholinergics in the treatment of neuroleptic side effects and are more sedating to boot. It is true that most over-the-counter sleep medications are antihistamines. They probably are at least mildly effective hypnotics and are not unreasonable choices in young, healthy patients. However, they are not as innocuous as they are commonly thought to be; older persons and others with neurological diseases are quite likely to experience side effects of hallucinosis or full-fledged delirium.

Disulfiram

Disulfiram (Antabuse) inhibits aldehyde dehydrogenase, which is involved in the metabolism of ethanol. The net result is that a person on the drug who ingests alcohol develops a reaction that may include nausea, vomiting, and (in more severe cases) seizures, cardiorespiratory collapse, and death. Antabuse has been used to treat alcohol dependence. It is not used widely, partly because of the medical risks of the reaction with alcohol, partly because some supervision is required to ensure daily compliance (otherwise the patient who wishes to resume drinking simply needs to stop the Antabuse for a few days), and partly because the only well designed study did not demonstrate much effectiveness.

Flumazenil

This benzodiazepine-receptor antagonist's main use is to acutely reverse the effects of benzodiazepine overdoses.

Methadone

This is an opioid with a long half-life and excellent bioavailability with oral dosing. It may be used to treat chronic pain, particularly in the terminally ill, having the advantage of any long–half-life opioid in offering continuous pain relief. Its half-life also offers advantages when using slow dosage reduction to withdraw patients safely from opioids. Finally, chronic administration of methadone as part of comprehensive outpatient drug dependence treatment ("methadone maintenance" programs) has clearly demonstrated effectiveness in reducing rates of relapse and improving function in patients with opioid dependence. (Such demonstrated usefulness has not, of course, prevented occasional public outcries about these programs; for this and many other reasons, funding for methadone treatment does not allow enough treatment slots to be available to meet all patients' needs.)

Opioid Antagonists

These agents block the action of opioids at the receptor level, hence the clever name for this category. Naloxone (Narcan) is given parenterally, is rapid but brief-acting, and is most useful for reversing acute symptoms of opioid intoxication (e.g., following overdose). Naltrexone (Trexan) is a long-acting oral agent. Studies of its use to prevent relapse in opioid dependence have been disappointing. However, it has been effective in treating alcohol dependence; why it decreases alcohol craving is not yet clear.

Tacrine

Optimistically given the brand name Cognex, tacrine is the first drug marketed in the U.S. for treatment of the cognitive deficits of Alzheimer's disease. Its main effects probably stem from promotion of central cholinergic activity via inhibition of acetylcholinesterase. Some studies suggest that tacrine can improve cognitive function in patients with Alzheimer's disease of mild to moderate severity. The clinical significance of this improvement, and consequently the role tacrine should or should not play in the routine management of this disease, remain unclear. Also, it is not known whether tacrine has any efficacy in more severely demented patients with Alzheimer's disease, or in patients with dementia of any severity from other causes.

Thyroid Hormones

There is considerable anecdotal evidence, and growing controlled evidence, that thyroid hormones may augment the efficacy of antidepressants and ECT in major depressive disorder, even in patients who are euthyroid to clinical examination and routine blood thyroid tests. Triiodothyronine (Cytomel) may be more effective than thyroxine (Synthroid). Thyroid supplementation may also be used to treat lithium-induced goiter (with or without concomitant hypothyroidism) if the benefit/risk ratio favors continued lithium treatment.

Zolpidem

Zolpidem (Ambien) is a newer hypnotic that has been heavily marketed as being a nonbenzodiazepine. Well, it is true that it is structurally not a benzodiazepine, but its mechanism of action appears to involve the benzodiazepine-GABA receptor complex. Extensive data have not yet been compiled, but there is no reason at this time to suppose that Ambien will be free of benzodiazepine side effects, including risk of dependence. Its half-life is reasonable for a hypnotic agent, so it may be a useful drug. But it probably does not have any real advantages over benzodiazepines, and it is more expensive.

ELECTROCONVULSIVE THERAPY

ECT has received an inordinate amount of bad press over the years, fostered by various elements of the mass media and by a small number of vocal people who claim to have had their lives ruined by it. Some part of this is deserved historically. More than 30 years ago, ECT administration was rather barbaric (patients were not given any anesthesia or sedation), and in the days before effective psychotropic medications or modern diagnostic classifications, ECT was used fairly indiscriminately.

But none of the bad press is deserved today. ECT is quite safe, enormously effective in certain well-defined clinical situations, and causes no permanent damage of any kind. Like any treatment modality, it has potential side effects, and benefits and risks must be discussed openly among clinicians, patients, and families before embarking on an ECT course.

Mechanism of Action

We don't know exactly how ECT works, any more than we know exactly how antidepressant medications work. We do know that it's the seizure that counts, and (probably) not the electricity. (Electrical stimulation is simply the safest and most reproducible way of inducing a controlled seizure.) We know that seizures are accompanied by an outpouring of catecholamines and many (most?) other neurotransmitters. We also know from animal models that a course of ECT results in longer-term changes, such as down regulation of beta-adrenergic receptors, which are similar to the longer-term changes seen with antidepressant medications.

Indications

ECT's efficacy is most clearly demonstrated for unipolar and bipolar depression, particularly for melancholic and psychotic subtypes. It is often reserved for patients who are unresponsive to or intolerant of medications. However, it may be a treatment of first choice for psychotic depression and for situations where the most rapid response is essential (e.g., a patient who is intractably suicidal or who requires nasogastric or IV fluids due to cessation of oral intake). Other indications for ECT include intractable mania, intractable psychotic symptoms in schizophrenia or schizoaffective disorder (especially if some affective symptoms are present), and catatonic syndromes. ECT also ameliorates the symptoms of Parkinson's disease, although it is not often used for this indication alone, partly because of high rates of rapid relapse.

Administration

ECT is typically given as a course of treatments. Increasingly, ECT is performed on an outpatient basis. The literature still fairly rages with debate about the optimal frequency of treatments, but in the U.S. the usual practice is three treatments per week. The course is continued until maximum benefit is reached or until side effects (usually cognitive) require slowing down or stopping the course. Most patients with depression require between 6 and 12 treatments, but this is quite variable. Some patients may achieve full remission or maximal improvement after 3 or 4 treatments, while others tolerate and achieve extra benefit from continuing through 15 or even 20 treatments.

After appropriate psychiatric and medical evaluations have ensured the indication and safety of the procedure, the patient gives informed consent. The patient is brought to the ECT treatment room, which is usually staffed by a psychiatric nurse and anesthesiologist along with the psychiatrist. The patient is anesthetized with an IV short-acting agent, usually a barbiturate (thiopental or methohexital), although propofol is gaining its proponents. Oxygen is administered by face mask, and the patient is ventilated ("bagged"). Succinylcholine is given IV, and the patient is monitored for maximum muscle paralysis by observing the depolarization-induced muscle fasciculations, and often by use of an electrical nerve stimulator. Then the ECT stimulus is given via electrodes placed on the scalp. ECT machines administer pulse-wave current for a brief duration (usually less than 1 second). Single-lead electroencephalography (EEG) and observation of tonic-clonic motor movements allow determination of seizure duration. With proper succinylcholine–induced paralysis, there is actually very little grossly observable muscle contraction, so usually a blood pressure cuff is inflated to greater than systolic pressure on one arm before the succinylcholine is given, enabling "unmodified" contractions to be visible in that extremity. The seizure typically lasts 30 to 45 seconds. The patient awakens rapidly after that and is allowed to resume independent ventilation. The whole procedure takes perhaps 5 minutes, after which the patient is monitored in a recovery area until full consciousness is regained. New trainees are inevitably disappointed by the lack of drama.

Although response rates to ECT are high (probably higher than for medication regimens), relapse is very likely unless continuation therapy is instituted. Usually this means beginning an appropriate medication shortly after the ECT course is completed. In patients who cannot tolerate or have failed all reasonable medication alternatives, continuation (and, for recurrent illness, long-term maintenance) ECT is used. Typically, this involves gradually decreasing the frequency of ECT, perhaps to once per week, then biweekly, then once per month indefinitely. Occasional patients may benefit from even less frequent ECT.

Side Effects

Because patients are anesthetized, they feel no pain and do not remember the treatment at all from the point at which the anesthetic is given. Some degree of grogginess is not uncommon for several hours after the treatment (although many persons do not experience this). On occasion, patients may be frankly delirious afterward; cognitive side effects may be cumulative, so delirium is more common later in a treatment course.

Other side effects are those common with anesthesia (although the seizure may contribute), including nausea and headache. Serious reactions to anesthetics are rare but possible. The risk of death during ECT is, if anything, lower than the mortality rate during other brief procedures using general anesthesia, which is considerably lower than the risk of death in the context of severe depressive states.

Although some patients escape significant cognitive side effects, many experience at least some degree of mental slowing and inefficiency during the ECT course. Some have more severe deficits in memory, attention, or other cognitive functions, which syndromically may manifest as delirium or dementia. These deficits resolve after discontinuing ECT, persisting, at the most, several weeks after the last treatment. Numerous studies have shown that there are *no* permanent cognitive or neuropsychological impairments caused by ECT. Neuroimaging studies have also failed to show any anatomic changes or lesions, even in patients who had received more than 100 treatments over their lifetime.

Cognitive deficits are neither associated with nor required for treatment response. Bilateral ECT (one electrode placed over each hemisphere) probably is more effective than unilateral ECT (both electrodes placed over the nondominant hemisphere), but bilateral ECT certainly is associated with greater cognitive side effects. Greater electric current, above the threshold for seizure induction, is also associated with more cognitive impairment. One well designed study noted that higher-dose (i.e., higher-current) unilateral treatment was more effective than lower-dose unilateral treatment, higher-dose bilateral was about equal in efficacy to lower-dose bilateral, and both of these were more effective than any unilateral treatment course.

LIGHT THERAPY

Phototherapy involves, unsurprisingly, exposure to bright lights. Typically, a room is equipped with special fluorescent lights that provide far more lux than ordinary indoor illumination. Patients sit in this room daily for treatments of 30 minutes or 1 hour. They are told not to stare at the lights but to allow their eyes to occasionally wander around the room (including over the lights).

The main indication for light therapy is major depressive disorder with a seasonal component. Light treatments may be the primary therapy or an adjunct to medications. The mechanism of action is not fully understood but is believed to involve the shifting of CNS circadian rhythms. Most patients respond better to treatments in the morning, but some have better response to late afternoon treatments; in practice, the most effective timing for a given patient is found empirically.

5

PART

Psychiatric Settings, Emergencies, and Special Topics

All the news that's fit to print—and that didn't fit in anywhere else.

17

CHAPTER

Where You'll Be Working and with Whom

Like most medical specialties, psychiatry is practiced in a wide variety of settings. Each serves its own patient population and is structured to meet the treatment needs and goals of that population. As a psychiatric trainee, you will draw on common core assessment skills when working in all sites but must learn how to focus your evaluations in relation to the setting. For example, detailed delineation of danger and acute symptoms is more important than obtaining a lengthy developmental history in the emergency room assessment of a patient brought by the police on mental hygiene arrest. Favored treatment modalities will also vary in relation to the setting's intended target patient population. Indeed, some treatments, such as group therapies aimed at specific problems (e.g., eating-disorder behaviors, substance-use troubles) may work best when they are embedded in the structure of a larger treatment program.

Ideally, you will be exposed to several settings during your rotation, giving you a better sense of the breadth of psychiatry than working in only one setting. Being in several settings will also give you an opportunity to define and refine your clinical skills as you learn which techniques are common across sites and which are limited to specific circumstances. In each site, ask yourself the following questions:

- What patient problems can and cannot be evaluated properly in this setting?
- What are the patient outcome goals of this setting?
- How does this setting relate to broader systems of psychiatric, medical, and other patient care?
- What is the role of the psychiatrist and of other disciplines in achieving the goals of this setting?

TREATMENT SETTINGS

Inpatient Psychiatric Units

Inpatient psychiatric units may exist in general (i.e., medical-surgical) hospitals. They also may be free-standing structures that are either privately owned or publicly funded (e.g., state mental hospitals). Most inpatient psychiatry units serve a general psychiatry population. Programs designed to target specific patients—by age, diagnosis, or other commonality (e.g., history of sexual abuse)—may exist on general units, or may be the sole offering of some subspecialty units.

Short-Term Units

Units may also be classified by average length of stay, with differences in patient populations and treatment goals. Short-term units are the most common. Various socioeconomic forces have converged to make longer-term units scarcer. Overall inpatient bed utilization is declining; patients who would have been hospitalized in the past are now being treated as outpatients. This means that the acuity level of the patients who *are* admitted has increased. Also, the average length of stay on general psychiatry short-term units has decreased over the past 10 years, from approximately 30 days to something approaching or reaching single digits! Debate still rages as to whether shorter length of stay leads to poorer quality of care. Early research suggests that short-term readmission rates are higher with shorter length of stay, but it is not clear if other measures of outcome are in fact worse.

Clearly, though, the *kind* of care offered has changed with the decreased length of stay. The emphasis is on identifying the patient's "focal problem," the reason the patient needed to be admitted in the first place. For example, while Mr. Tetris' primary *diagnosis* is major depression, his *focal problem* is suicidal ideation. As soon as his suicidality is reduced enough that he can be safely managed as an outpatient, he will be discharged to outpatient care, whether or not the major depression is resolved. Other examples of inpatient-level focal problems include homicidality (if caused by a mental disorder) and inadvertent danger to self (e.g., patients who are unable to feed, dress, or otherwise care for themselves because of psychotic disorganization).

Once the focal problem is identified, the inpatient team addresses it accordingly. To do so requires careful psychiatric and medical evaluation. This involves determination of diagnoses and implementation of appropriate treatments. It also involves understanding the patient's social environment, including supports and stressors, in order to intervene effectively. In practice, treatments begun on the inpatient unit may include:

- Somatic therapies (i.e., medications or electroconvulsive therapy [ECT]).
- Individual psychotherapy, which will typically be focused on "here and now" issues including psychoeducation (helping the patient understand his or her illness, its implications, and the need for treatment) and crisis-oriented supportive psychotherapy.
- Group work, or involvement in the unit "milieu." Highly structured, task-oriented groups are most useful for patients at a lower functional level (e.g., acutely psychotic or disorganized patients), while talk-oriented therapy groups with a focus on short-term issues are aimed at higher-functioning patients.
- Family work, which may include data gathering, providing support and psychoeducation, and crisis-oriented therapy to promote symptom reduction in the patient and the family and encourage family support of the recommended discharge plan.
- Liaison with previous or future outpatient treaters, caregivers, or social agencies, with the aims of data gathering, psychoeducation, and solidification of a discharge plan that provides for the patient's needs.

To accomplish all these tasks rapidly and efficiently usually requires the coordinated efforts of a multidisciplinary treatment team, as discussed later in this chapter. In most inpatient units, the psychiatrist is the nominal "captain" of the team, with ultimate responsibility for proper diagnosis and treatment plan implementation. However, precise distribution of role responsibilities varies widely in different units and professional communities.

Long-Term Units

Long-term units encompass a variety of patient populations. Depending on the patients served, length of stay may average several weeks, several months, or several years, although the latter has become rather rare in the current socioeconomic climate. Typically, patients are admitted to long-term units only after failing multiple attempts at conventional therapies, which may have included several short-term hospitalizations along with attempts at outpatient treatment. Their conditions, then, are often marked by chronicity, treatment refractoriness, noncompliance, or several psychiatric or substance-use comorbidities.

Long-term units tend to be free-standing rather than based in general hospitals. *Private long-term hospitals* tend to have patients from higher socioeconomic strata, since health insurance plans often do not pay for these stays. Patients may have intractable psychotic disorders such as schizophrenia. Others may have severe personality disorders with comorbid mood, anxiety, or substance-use disorders. Some specialized programs may cater to other specific diagnoses, such as severe and chronic eating disorders or posttraumatic stress disorder (PTSD).

Publicly funded long-term units serve many patients with few socioeconomic resources, which may contribute to or be the result of their psychopathology. (See the section later in this chapter on Systems of Care.) Patients in state mental hospital long-term units mostly have chronic psychotic disorders such as severe, intractable schizophrenia or schizoaffective disorder. Some patients may have particularly chronic or disabling forms of mood disorders, "organic" mental disorders, or other conditions. Other publicly funded units vary in patient composition depending on their referral sources. For example, it should be no surprise that Veterans Affairs hospital units have many patients with combat-related PTSD, which may be comorbid with substance use, personality disorders, or other psychiatric pathologies.

Patients who make it to long-term units generally have failed to improve with several attempts at somatic therapies and brief psychotherapies. Therefore, along with continued attention to relevant somatic therapies, the emphasis on long-term units is on more intensive psychotherapies. Theoretical orientations of this work may include rehabilitative (e.g., teaching social and vocational skills to patients disabled with schizophrenia), exploratory psychodynamic, or behavioral treatments, depending on the patients served and the traditions of the institution. Most experienced clinicians do believe that such long-term work is helpful for carefully selected patients, but there are few empirical data to guide psychotherapeutic approaches in such complex, often multi-disordered clinical situations. Some institutions offer intensive individual psychotherapy, which may include two, three, or more sessions per week. Most long-term units are also built around the therapeutic milieu, with group therapies and activities forming a major part of the treatment plan. Many also address longer-term family issues in ongoing family therapies.

Partial Hospitals and Day Treatment Programs

The array of intensive outpatient programs available to patients may at first appear bewildering. These programs differ from traditional office-based outpatient practices in that they offer a half day or full day of treatment modalities, and patients may attend the program several days per week. Although the distinctions at times are somewhat arbitrary, let us divide these programs into two main types: partial-hospital and day-treatment programs.

Partial Hospitals

These programs usually aim to treat acutely ill patients, often helping to avert or shorten inpatient hospitalization. The level of multidisciplinary staffing is typically close to that of an inpatient unit. Patients often attend a full day's program 5 days per week, with some decrease in the frequency of attendance as they improve and prepare for discharge from the partial hospital. Most programs have a target or maximum length of stay, which helps both the patient and the treatment team focus on achievable short-term goals. Partial hospitals may be free-standing entities or may be located in a general or psychiatric hospital. Increasingly, partial hospitals have close administrative or physical ties with inpatient units and less intensive outpatient sites as part of a comprehensive system of care to encompass fluctuations in the severity of patients' disorders.

Partial hospitals usually emphasize group activities and therapies, but also provide close attention to somatic therapies and employ individual and family work as well. Given the high level of staffing, including psychiatrists, the eligibility and diagnostic criteria for admission to these programs are quite similar to those for inpatient admission. Patients do need to be safe enough—that is, not imminently dangerous to themselves or others—to go home at the end of the day. They also must have the means and the desire to come to the program, since staff members cannot force them to attend. Most partial hospitals are open to general psychiatric patients, although some may be specialty-oriented.

Day Treatment Programs

Structurally, day-treatment programs are less intensive versions of partial hospitals. They may have lower staff-to-patient ratios and fewer psychiatrists (and general medical personnel) available, at least partly accounting for the even more prominent role of groups in most day-treatment programs. Some or all patients may be expected to come for shorter days or for fewer days per week. Clearly, then, day programs are not designed to handle the level of psychiatric acuity found in partial hospitals or short-term inpatient hospitals. Rather, their goal is often more analogous to the rehabilitative aims of long-term inpatient units. The lower day-to-day intensity of treatment is counterbalanced by the leverages afforded by time, since most day programs have considerably longer lengths of stay than partial hospitals (many weeks to months), and some allow patients to have indefinite "residence." This time allows the patient and treatment team to address long-standing problems with interpersonal relatedness, family issues, or other social needs. The structure of the program may be useful for patients who are unable to create such a socially supportive structure in their own lives but who function well when provided with one.

Because of the nature of longer-term outpatient work, day-treatment programs are more likely to be specialized, that is, to target patients with particular diagnoses or treatment needs. After all, the ongoing psychotherapeutic and social needs of patients with severe schizophrenia are quite different from, say, those of alcohol-dependent patients with PTSD. It is difficult, then, to comment usefully here about the details of day-treatment program structure since variation is the norm.

Outpatient Settings

More and more trainees on psychiatric rotations are gaining exposure to practice in a variety of outpatient settings. This is all to the good, as it allows you to see patients with major psychopathology during periods of relative symptomatic improvement as well as patients with less disabling disorders whom you might never encounter in inpatient, partial hospital, or other acute settings.

Unfortunately, the very breadth of practice types and patients served makes it hard to say much that is useful here other than to recognize that such diversity does exist. Sources of this variability include:

- *Site*, e.g., hospital-based clinic, free-standing private or public mental health clinic, private office, home visits ("house calls" are enjoying a minor resurgence in psychiatry, as in general medicine)
- *Practice staff structure*, e.g., solo psychiatrist, psychiatrist group (akin to models of group coverage in general medicine), multidisciplinary team
- *Clinical problems encountered*, e.g., open, general psychiatric practice versus practice limited to certain diagnoses ("Mood Disorders Clinic") versus practice limited to patients who might benefit from specific treatment modalities ("Behavioral Therapy Center")
- *Types of services offered*, e.g., consultation, crisis intervention, short-term or long-term psychotherapy, ongoing "medication management" without formal psychotherapy, in-

dividual, family, or group psychotherapies. Most sites offer some combination of the foregoing, depending on clinical needs

- *Length of patient visits,* e.g., quarter hour (used for brief follow-ups of known patients), half hour (lengthier follow-ups, some forms of psychotherapy with selected patients), hour (most traditional psychotherapies), longer visits (extensive evaluations, some crisis interventions)
- *Frequency of patient visits,* e.g., weekly (most psychotherapies and acute illness management), two or more times per week (intensive exploratory long-term psychotherapy or psychoanalysis, severe acuity/crisis management), biweekly or less often (patients who are improving or stable)
- *Availability of procedures,* e.g., physical evaluations (from simple orthostatic vital signs checks to full work-ups), phlebotomy, electrocardiograms, light therapy, outpatient ECT

Consultation Services

The pathognomonic feature, so to speak, of consulting work involves the essence of the psychiatrist's relationship to the patient. In most other circumstances, the patient (with or without his or her family) is clearly the person being served, and the psychiatrist has ultimate responsibility to educate and otherwise intervene with the patient. In a psychiatric consultation, the ultimate responsibility rests with the referring physician or provider. The psychiatrist is, in a sense, serving the patient indirectly by serving the referring doctor—that is, by using specialty expertise to answer the referral questions.

This arrangement, while often enormously useful, sometimes clouds the nature of the psychiatrist-patient relationship, particularly if the consultant comes to assume some ongoing responsibility for the patient's treatment. As in the rest of medicine, when several subspecialists are involved, it is crucial to make it clear to the patient and to all the caregivers who has the overall responsibility and authority for the patient's care. Certain pieces of this responsibility may be delegated to expert consultants, but the details of this delegation must be as explicit as possible to work smoothly. For example, it may be arranged for the psychiatric "consultant" to see the patient regularly for psychotherapy and psychotropic medication recommendations, while the primary care physician manages the remainder of the patient's disorders and medications and also remains aware of the psychiatric assessments and treatments.

Questions to Consider

Since the consultant's true "client" is the referring caregiver, several points should be considered beyond the clinical evaluation of the patient in question:

Who really wanted the consultation? Usually the answer is straightforward: The referring physician wanted the consultation! Occasionally, though, the official referring person is not primarily invested in your consultation. The request may have been prompted by other providers (other consultants, residents, medical students, nursing staff), social workers (who may hope that a psychiatric consultation will expedite their efforts regarding patient disposition), the patient's family, or the patient himself or herself. Understanding where the consult was generated will help you answer the important questions below, and help you direct your recommendations most helpfully.

Now that you know who referred the patient,

what do you know about the referrer? The point here is that the more you know *about* the referrer and the more of an ongoing relationship you have with him or her, the better you'll be able to figure out the implicit questions (see below) and respond to them appropriately. What are the relative strengths and limitations of this person's knowledge and skills in psychiatric issues? What are his or her attitudes toward mental disorders, psychiatry in general, and you in particular? Some settings establish formal administrative structures linking psychiatric consultants with referrers, which are known as liaison arrangements. However, liaison-type work happens with all effective psychiatric consultation, creating the framework and interpersonal relationships that make the consultations more helpful to referrers and patients alike.

What is the **explicit** *reason for the consultation?* It is extremely important to ask referrers to identify what they want you to do. Sometimes the request is necessarily broad or vague, such as, "I know the patient is in emotional distress, but I don't know what it is. Please do a diagnostic assessment." Dialogue between you and the referrer may narrow the focus a bit, to something like "Please evaluate this patient's suicidal ideation," "Recommend an antidepressant," "Evaluate the patient's capacity to refuse medical treatment," or "Recommend treatment to reduce the patient's agitation." Of course, in your evaluation of the patient you will need to think more broadly; just because the referrer asked you to recommend an antidepressant doesn't mean that you will consider only depression in your differential diagnosis, or that you will consider only antidepressants as therapeutic options. But knowing the explicit question gives you some focus to begin with, and something to respond to, to satisfactorily aid the referrer. For example, if you choose *not* to recommend an antidepressant, you will need to explain explicitly why not, in addition to explaining whatever you do recommend.

What are the **implicit** *reasons for the consultation?* Asking this question means addressing the process as well as the content of the consultation. Admittedly, there are many times when there are no implicit or hidden reasons for the consult. Yet it is important to look carefully for such behind-the-scenes dynamics. When they arise, particularly with psychiatric issues, they are often quite affect-laden, and must be directly addressed to complete the consultation satisfactorily. For example, a medical team asks you in an open-ended fashion to evaluate a patient's capacity to refuse treatment. It is likely that the team has its own opinion (or sometimes mutually opposing opinions) about the patient's capacity, as well as any of several strong affects regarding this patient who is refusing their recommendations. If your opinion about the patient's capacity differs from what the team expects or wishes you to indicate, careful explanation, discussion, and other liaison-type interactions may be needed to help the team accept your opinion and implement the appropriate treatment plan. If the team members are divided among themselves, your consultation may extend to helping them resolve their own conflicts to best serve the patient's interest.

Consultation Settings

Psychiatrists may offer consultation services in many settings, including:

- *Inpatient general hospital floors,* the most common setting for academic/teaching consultation services.
- *Outpatient primary care or specialty clinics or*

services (e.g., dialysis units). The psychiatrist may see the patients "on site" (i.e., at the clinic), or in the psychiatrist's own office.

- *Outpatient private practices.* Most commonly, the patient is seen in the psychiatrist's own office, but on-site consultation is becoming more popular.
- *Residential settings* (nursing homes, adult care facilities, group homes, etc.).
- *Forensic settings* (prisons, court-related consultations, attorney- or insurance company–requested consultations related to legal actions or disability claims).
- *Employers.* Companies may request consultation services on an individual basis for specific employees or on a group basis for more global occupational difficulties. (This latter is most often performed by occupational psychologists.) In one interesting example described in the New England Journal of Medicine a number of years ago, a psychiatrist consulted to a professional football team that was having morale and leadership difficulties along with poor performance on the playing field. The psychiatrist used techniques derived from group psychotherapy and, of course, went on to report how well the team did in the playoffs the next year. . . .

Psychiatric Emergency Rooms

As with other emergency rooms (ERs), the psychiatric emergency room's main functions are to assess all comers, initiate emergent-level treatments, and link up the patients with appropriate subsequent services ranging from inpatient admissions to outpatient treatments to a variety of other dispositions (including no treatment at all). Thus, the main psychiatric skills used are diagnostic and situational assessment techniques. Crisis interventions—medications, individual, or family psychotherapies—are often employed to improve the patient's clinical state and allow the use of the least restrictive means of care appropriate (e.g., avoiding an inpatient stay when possible). As a trainee in the "psych ER" (or "EW" or "ED," or whatever your hospital calls it), you will have an opportunity to hone these skills.

Also, as with other parts of the ER, the open door policy of the setting invites an enormous range of patients and patient problems. This offers you a wonderful exposure to broad clinical material. As well, unlike most of the patients you will encounter in other settings, many of the patients in the ER have never been diagnosed or treated psychiatrically before, giving you an unparalleled opportunity to exercise independent thinking as you formulate the cases.

The types of problems and situations you'll encounter can never be reduced to a simple list, but will include:

- True psychiatric emergencies: suicidal ideation, homicidal ideation, and so on (see Chap. 18)
- Acute exacerbations of major mental disorders: acute psychosis, mania, severe depression, often in the course of related Axis II disorders
- Substance use–related syndromes: intoxication; withdrawal; substance-induced mood, psychotic, or other disorders; drug-seeking behavior, such as patients asking for pain medications or hypnotics
- New-onset psychiatric symptoms of major or less major proportions: all of the above, plus anxiety and cognitive deficit syndromes (in less severe cases, the ER essentially

serves as a diagnostic and triage center for outpatient care)

- Other secondary psychiatric syndromes: That is, medical illnesses that present with prominent behavioral symptoms, leading to triage to the psychiatric part of the ER
- Consultations to the medical/surgical ER: problems that present a mixture of the above plus the concerns previously discussed under "Consultation Services"

SYSTEMS OF CARE

In the course of their work, psychiatrists may intersect with a variety of systems of care. These systems are typically composed of several treatment settings that are theoretically closely linked, so that patients served by each system can move easily through different levels or types of care as their condition warrants. Some of the more widely prevalent systems are described here.

Health Maintenance Organizations

By definition, patients insured by health maintenance organizations (HMOs) may see only HMO-participating providers. Only some HMOs offer a well-integrated system of care to patients in need of psychiatric services. Most have caps on mental health utilization. Examples include setting a maximum number of outpatient psychiatric visits covered per year or a maximum number of psychiatric inpatient days per year (or per lifetime). Many HMOs use partial hospital days toward the inpatient cap, at ratios such as two partial for one inpatient hospital day. For office visits, some HMOs use a clinic model, in which patients primarily see less expensive, nonphysician therapists for intakes and ongoing psychotherapy, while psychiatrists provide backup consultation regarding medications, diagnostic issues, and the shape of the overall treatment plan. HMOs and managed care systems clearly do reduce mental health expenditures in the short run. Many have argued that the quality and quantity of care offered are considerably less than ideal. Others note that the cost savings may be illusory, since patients with untreated or poorly treated mental disorders have higher utilization of general medical resources. Also, most HMO systems tend not to be geared toward patients with severe, debilitating mental disorders, many of whom lack the resources to pay for private insurance.

Severely and Persistently Mentally Ill

The severely and persistently mentally ill (SPMI) population includes persons with chronic psychotic disorders (primarily schizophrenia), along with malignant, treatment-refractory, debilitating forms of mood, personality, or other disorders. By definition, these patients as a group tend to have high rates of psychiatric hospitalization and to need highly structured, intensive, long-term psychiatric treatments and psychosocial rehabilitation. Systems of care for this population must therefore include access to inpatient units, short-term and long-term partial hospitals and day programs, clinics, and a wide array of ancillary services including social work, occupational and activities therapies, vocational rehabilitation, and so forth. An additional strategy is the use of intensive case management, which allocates specified staff to have low-volume, high-intensity case loads, enabling them to spend the time needed to stay in touch with noncompliant or recalcitrant patients (by visiting them in their homes if necessary) and to provide transportation, meals, or other access to whatever the patients need.

Needless to say, this wide range of intensive services is expensive. Often much of the front-line care is provided by nonphysician (i.e., less expensive) professionals. Psychiatrists usually conduct diagnostic evaluations at intake, initiate and monitor somatic therapies, and supervise treatment plans, including the progress of psychosocial therapies.

Also, since these services are expensive, and the patients are usually too impaired to hold steady jobs and have private health insurance, most SPMI systems depend largely or entirely on public support. This support includes both federal and state monies, through programs such as Medicaid. Distribution and allocation of funds takes place at the state level, which makes current SPMI systems thematically (and sometimes literally) the direct descendant of the days when huge state hospitals housed many thousands of chronically mentally ill patients. In principle, the money that once paid for long-term inpatient care has been shifted to provide for the array of outpatient services discussed above, although in practice the funds available are prone to budget-cutting efforts in state legislatures. Some states have a system of separate state hospitals and outpatient programs (community mental health centers); others pay private health care organizations and university medical centers to provide these services for indigent patients.

Substance Dependence

Systems of care for patients with substance-use disorders exist in a parallel universe to the rest of mental health services. This universe has numerous points of intersection with the psychiatry universe, but it is an autonomous domain nonetheless. The substance-dependence system provides for safe management of acute withdrawal from alcohol and other drugs (detox) and also includes inpatient, partial hospital and day programs, and traditional outpatient models of treating drug dependency.

Why such a parallel system? Part of the reason relates to extrinsic factors, including the historical development of addiction treatment separate from both insane asylums (which treated the severely mentally ill) and nonasylum psychiatrists (who earlier this century tended to treat solely healthier ambulatory patients). Another extrinsic factor is payment mechanisms, since insurance coverage and other (e.g., governmental) funding sources are allocated separately for addictions and other mental illnesses. Intrinsic factors related to treatment methods also play a role in the separation of the systems. Since treatment goals for most mental disorders include fostering the patient's autonomy and sense of responsibility for his or her own actions and life, psychiatric treatments tend to require trust in the patient and family to carry through on their share of the treatment burden, such as taking prescribed medications and working actively in psychotherapies. By contrast, because of the nature of substance-use disorders (and the high comorbidity of antisocial behaviors and personality disorders), addiction treatments tend to assume that the patient is going to be untruthful to the treater at times. Harsh and direct confrontation, routine breathalyzer or urine toxicology screens, linking privileges (e.g., limits to leave the hospital, getting a weekend's supply of methadone) tightly to behavior—all these techniques are prominent parts of most treatment plans for drug dependence and all are somewhat antithetical to the traditional spirit or practice of the rest of psychiatry. It is no surprise, then, that separate systems arose to administer these different kinds of interventions.

Unfortunately for those who prefer neat and clean divisions of labor, comorbidity of substance-use disorders and SPMIs such as schizophrenia has become extremely prevalent over the past 15 years or so. This is at least partially coincident with the rise in crack cocaine use in the poor urban areas where many patients with SPMIs live. Attempts to treat these "dually diagnosed" or "MICA" (**M**entally **I**ll **C**hemical **A**busers) patients didn't work very well in most previously existing settings: The addictions programs dealt poorly with acute psychosis or suicidal ideation, while the psychiatric programs dealt poorly with the substance use, which would exacerbate both psychotic symptoms and medication noncompliance. Consequently, many large psychiatric systems of care, especially SPMI programs in recent years, have created specialized MICA programs that blend both addiction and psychiatric treatment approaches, allowing more successful care of these patients.

One additional point regarding systems of care for drug dependence: Self-help groups such as Alcoholics Anonymous, Narcotics Anonymous, and various other 12-step programs exist in abundance in most American communities. They can be of enormous benefit for many patients. For some they may be the sole treatment required to achieve sobriety and rebuild social and occupational stability. For others a combination of self-help and professional addictions treatment is most effective. In recent years the attitudes of addictions professionals and self-help movement leaders have become more accepting of the usefulness of such combined approaches.

Mental Retardation/Developmental Disabilities

Public funds support the educational and residential care needs of people with significant mental retardation or developmental disabilities (MRDD) such as autism. Again, although these disorders are defined in the *Diagnostic and Statistical Manual of Mental Disorders* (DSM-IV) as mental disorders, a combination of historical, financial, and clinical issues resulted in the creation of a system separate from traditional child or adult psychiatric treatment systems. However, other psychiatric symptoms (e.g., depression, psychosis) and behavioral disturbances (e.g., self-injurious actions, aggressivity) frequently coexist with MRDD. These manifestations may be treatable in traditional psychiatric settings in patients with borderline intellectual functioning or mild mental retardation. For those with more severe MRDD-spectrum illness, care is usually best provided by ongoing psychiatric consultation-liaison to the MRDD facilities within which the patient lives or works. Again, funding for such consultation is often fragile, depending as it does on state or other governmental budgets.

Nursing Homes and Other Geriatric Residential Care

Chapter 19 will discuss psychiatric issues in the elderly at somewhat greater length. We'll just note here that chronic debilitating mental disorders, including psychiatric disturbances associated with dementing illnesses such as Alzheimer's disease, are quite common in older persons. In decades past, many of the most behaviorally disturbed demented elderly resided in state mental institutions. In recent years, deinstitutionalization has drastically shrunk the number of such patients in state hospitals. As a result, these patients end up being cared for at home or in residences originally designed for the physically disabled, such as nursing homes and adult care facilities. In other words, these facilities have become the de facto state hospital system for the chronically mentally ill elderly. Psychiatric consultation-liaison services are required to successfully address such patients' needs in these settings.

MULTIDISCIPLINARY ROLES AND TEAMS

While many private psychiatric practices may operate solely with psychiatrists, most other treatment settings are staffed by a variety of professionals. The roles of these professionals may vary from one setting to another and also may overlap to some extent. To a trainee new to psychiatry, this profusion of disciplines and roles may seem confusing, and the role of the physician may appear to be less clear-cut than in other medical specialties. Yet you will find that other professionals have much to offer you in your educational experience. At the same time, psychiatric physicians do have well-defined roles in each setting, which will become apparent to you as you gain knowledge and experience in the field. This section will discuss briefly the backgrounds and roles of some of the professionals you will encounter.

Psychiatrists

Psychiatrists are physicians with specialty residency training in the diagnosis and treatment of patients with mental disorders. Their training includes at least 4 years of residency after medical school. Typically, the PGY-1 (internship) year consists of at least 4 to 6 months of medicine, pediatrics, or other nonpsychiatric services, with the rest of the year usually including neurology as well as psychiatry rotations. Many complete a full year of residency on nonpsychiatric services. The remaining years of residency include exposure to psychiatric inpatient, outpatient, emergency room, and consultation settings. Seminars cover a wide range of basic and applied topics, while intensive one-to-one faculty clinical supervision helps develop individual, family, and group psychotherapy abilities along with diagnostic and psychopharmacological skills.

The psychotherapeutic skills of psychiatrists are not unique; other professionals are able to deliver quality psychotherapy. However, psychiatrists are specifically skilled regarding diagnosis (particularly in relation to medical illnesses that may be comorbid with, or contributory to, the psychopathology) and the development of biopsychosocial treatment plans including somatic therapies. In most academic medical centers, psychiatrists are more or less the "captains" of the multidisciplinary treatment team and have ultimate attending-level responsibility for their patients. In many other settings, psychiatrists play a consulting role to other mental health professionals who are the primary treatment providers. (Sometimes this role is termed "medical backup," although many believe this phrase is inappropriate.)

Psychologists

Some psychologists are trained at the master's degree level. These persons are typically employed as psychotherapists, either in private practices or in clinic or other group multidisciplinary settings. However, most psychologists that you are likely to encounter in academic settings have doctorate-level training, either a PhD in psychology or PsyD (doctor of psychology) degree. (We will speak here of clinical psychologists; experimental psychologists do not see or treat patients but conduct research ranging from molecular biology to animal or human subject work.) PsyD training includes both classroom and clinical work and is strongly oriented toward developing the skills and knowledge needed for clinical practice. PhD training includes classroom, clinical, and research experiences. This education includes much deeper and broader exposure to the basic sciences of psychology and to research methodologies than most physicians obtain during their undergraduate or postgraduate medical training. The combination of psychological and methodological training make psychologists qualified to administer and interpret psychological testing (see Chap. 13).

Clinical experiences of doctorate psychology trainees vary widely. Some rotate through academic psychiatry settings and therefore develop diagnostic and treatment planning skills analogous to those of psychiatrists. Their skills are analogous but not identical because psychologists draw on their more extensive education in psychological sciences but do not have medical training, cannot diagnose or treat comorbid medical conditions, and cannot prescribe medications or administer ECT. Other psychology graduate students may not train in psychiatric settings, but gain experience and skills in administering outpatient psychotherapies (individual, group, or family) or using psychological skills in nonpatient settings (e.g., corporate psychology).

Psychologists may serve many roles in multidisciplinary psychiatric clinical settings. Some of these roles may be quite focused, such as providing psychotherapy or psychological testing. Other roles may be broader, including leading treatment teams, clinics, or units.

Nurses

Staff registered nurses in inpatient units or in partial hospital or day treatment programs are responsible for management of the overall milieu, including issues of patient safety (suicidal ideation and aggressivity). They provide careful, trained observations of patients' behaviors and interpersonal interactions, using these data to collaborate with other multidisciplinary treatment team members to help make diagnostic assessments, implement therapeutic interventions, and monitor patient response. Nurses also may participate in family meetings and lead unit groups. Also, they are responsible for physical care assessments and interventions similar to nursing roles on general medical units.

Nurses at the master's degree level have additional training in psychiatric diagnosis and in psychotherapies. They may offer psychotherapy independently in private practice or may evaluate and treat patients in multidisciplinary settings such as clinics. In some communities, psychiatric nurse practitioners, who have additional training in diagnosis and therapeutics (including psychopharmacology), have limited prescription privileges and can function with a greater degree of autonomy, again analogous to the role of nurse practitioners in general medical settings.

Social Workers

In addition to the standard training received by all social workers (which may include bachelor's,

master's, or higher-level degrees), psychiatric social workers have additional educational experiences related to psychopathology and psychotherapies. In multidisciplinary academic medical
center settings, the social workers typically take a
prominent role in involving families in patients'
treatments. This may include obtaining history
from collateral informants, and leading or co-
leading family meetings that offer psychoeducation or other psychotherapeutic interventions.
Unit groups may be led by social work staff. Social workers are also usually responsible for liaison with community agencies to access resources
and implement optimal discharge planning. This
often requires developing and maintaining relationships with relevant systems of care external to
their own unit.

In private practice, psychiatric social workers,
particularly those with master's level or higher
training, may offer a wide variety of psychotherapies, including individual work. Many social
workers' interests and practices tend to emphasize family or group therapies.

Activities Therapists

Multidisciplinary treatment settings often employ persons with training in specialized fields
such as recreational, art, or music therapy. These
varied treatment modalities, which are usually
used in groups but may also be applied to individual work, are designed to assess and develop
psychosocial, cognitive, and physical skills. Activities therapists may also lead other unit
groups and work with other members of the
treatment team to manage the unit milieu and
implement individualized patient treatment
plans.

Some therapists with these specialized backgrounds may see patients privately for ongoing therapy. Often the goals of such therapies are analogous to the goals of other longer-term psychotherapies, using modalities such as art or music to facilitate expression of thoughts and affects and to serve as a vehicle for the development of a therapeutic alliance with the therapist.

Therapists with other backgrounds, such as occupational or physical therapy, may usefully aid in the assessment or treatment of psychiatric patients, particularly geriatric patients and SPMI patients who need longer-term psychosocial rehabilitation.

Paraprofessionals

Psychiatric techicians ("psych techs") and nursing assistants may play a prominent role in patient care, especially in acute hospital settings. Their educational backgrounds and work experience may vary, depending on the requirements of the employing institution. Typically, paraprofessionals work closely with nursing staff to manage the unit milieu, help implement psychiatric treatment plans, and provide needed physical care.

18

CHAPTER

Psychiatric Emergencies

This chapter will consider several topics, linked only by their potential for acuteness.

SUICIDE

Suicidality exists on a continuum of self-destructive behaviors, from chronic acts that may ultimately prove harmful (e.g., cigarette smoking), to physically harmful acute acts without intent or potential of death, to acts with clear intent or potential of killing oneself.

The term suicide "gesture" is sometimes used to refer to suicide attempts of low lethality. Beware, though: Use of this expression often says as much about our own reaction to the attempt (and the attempter) as it does about the objective reality of the event. Examples of low-lethality suicide attempts include superficial cutting, burning (e.g., with a lit cigarette), or swallowing objects (e.g., tacks, paper clips). Sometimes the motive for these acts is external and obvious, such as avoiding prison. Other patients describe these acts as means of relieving tension or anxiety. Occasionally, psychotic patients use such behaviors to try to maintain contact with reality—the reality being the pain or wound that ensues—or as a distraction from their internal psychotic preoccupations. In any case, motives are difficult to discern reliably. Self-destructive acts should *always* be taken seriously.

Clinical Risk Factors

Suicide attempters and completers are different, if overlapping, populations. Some of their risk factors and clinical characteristics are similar, and others are quite different. For example, rates of suicide attempts are high among young adult females, which contrasts with the demographic profile of suicides (discussed below). As another example, suicide attempts may be common among persons with severe personality disorders—indeed, they are part of the criteria set for borderline personality disorder—but personality pathology alone accounts for only a small portion of completed suicides.

Factors related to completed suicide include:

- Older age: Suicide in adolescents gets far more press, partly because adolescent suicide rates have been rising, and partly because suicide is one of the top causes of death in this age group. Suicide rates, however, are much higher in the elderly. In addition to their greater frailty, older people are much more likely to use highly lethal means when they try to take their lives, making the ratio of completers to attempters higher than in younger people.
- Male gender: Males of all ages are more

likely to use violent and lethal means, again raising their rate of completed suicide.

- Caucasian race: The higher suicide rates found in U.S. whites, as compared with other ethnicities, no doubt reflect a complex combination of factors.
- Other demographic and cultural factors: Suicide rates vary greatly across religious groups, nationalities, and other cultural markers. Suicide is also associated with living alone; widowed, divorced or separated marital status; and unemployment or retirement. These latter factors may contribute to suicide directly or may themselves be manifestations of the clinical conditions that predispose to suicide.
- Psychiatric diagnoses: Most, but by no means all, persons who kill themselves have a diagnosable psychiatric disorder at the time of their death. The most common diagnostic categories include chronic psychotic disorders (e.g., schizophrenia, schizoaffective disorder), substance-use disorders (especially alcohol dependence), and mood disorders (mostly major depression). In the suicidal elderly, mood disorders clearly predominate among those with a diagnosable condition.
- Stressors: Stressful life events are clearly risk factors for suicide. Common events or themes include interpersonal or other losses, medical illnesses (actual and perceived), and family discord.
- Personality: Diagnoses of *Diagnostic and Statistical Manual of Mental Disorders* (DSM-IV) personality disorders are of limited usefulness in predicting suicide, but empirical research has begun to support clinical notions that suicidal persons have rigid, inflexible, or otherwise limited coping mecha-

nisms, particularly in their approach to problem solving.

Additional Perspectives on Suicidal Behavior

Attempts to understand the biopsychosocial pathophysiology of suicidal behavior have drawn on numerous levels of conceptual organization. All may play some role, although the predominant factors may vary among different suicidal people. We cannot do justice here to the breadth and depth of the field of suicidology. We have already alluded to theories involving personality, stressors, cultural factors, other social factors, and the biopsychosocial concomitants of gender and age. Three additional, overlapping perspectives are worth highlighting here.

1. There may be a genetics, neurobiology, and neuroendocrinology of suicide that cuts across psychiatric diagnostic boundaries. For example, suicidal persons may have decreased activity of serotonergic systems, analogous to (but independent of) the decrease seen in depression.
2. Suicidal behavior may have any of several overt or unconscious "goals," including expressions of :
   a. Despair (the desire to remove oneself from the environment).
   b. Rage (the desire to express anger or exact punishment on others).
   c. Help-seeking (the desire to change the behavior of others to get one's own needs met).
3. In some cases, suicidality may be helpfully understood as nothing more or less than a symptom of an acute Axis I disorder, which will remit when the acute episode remits. This

perspective does not always apply, but it is useful in many clinical situations.

Assessment

In assessing suicidality, one must consider the following factors:

- The demographic and clinical risk factors listed previously
- Explicit delineation of the patient's ideation, plans, and intent, as discussed in Chapter 12
- Details of the attempt itself: the extent of advance preparations (such as completion of a will, shifting bank accounts for one's heirs, and so forth), precautions taken to preclude discovery, and the lethality of the method
- The patient's degree of hopelessness (the single symptom that may be the best correlate of suicide risk)

It is important to be humble about our ability to predict suicide, which is an extraordinarily complex, multidetermined behavior. It is also a relatively unlikely outcome in any single given clinical situation. Therefore, even the most sophisticated attempts to develop predictive algorithms, using as rich a clinical database as possible, have failed to predict suicide with enough accuracy to be clinically helpful. We do know much with which to inform our clinical judgment, but the "judgment" part remains.

VIOLENCE

Violence is, of course, an increasingly prominent and problematic part of our society. While the neurobiologic, psychological, and social sciences can help us understand violent behavior better, psychiatry as a clinical discipline—that is, the medical specialty of diagnosing and treating mental disorders—can offer only limited insights and is even more limited in its ability to predict or prevent specific acts of violence.

Much of the psychiatric assessment of patients for violence entirely overlaps with the general assessments discussed previously. Much of the larger consideration of violent behavior is beyond the scope of this book. What follows are a few additional pointers of relevance to your work in clinical settings.

Clinical Risk Factors

The following are useful clinical guides rather than statements about absolute risk. For example, in the community psychotic persons may not be at any greater risk of violent acts than the general population, but in psychiatric or other patient care settings, psychosis may lead to violence and is worth noting as part of your clinical assessment.

- Male gender
- Prior history of violence
- Prior history of, or current evidence for, other types of poor impulse control
- Psychiatric diagnosis or acute state, including:
  - Mania (may be the single best predictor of violence in psychiatric inpatient settings)
  - Psychosis
  - Substance-related states, particularly intoxications and withdrawals
  - Cognitive impairments, including delirium, dementia, and mental retardation
  - Personality disorders (particularly those marked by chronic difficulties with im-

pulse control, such as borderline or anti-social personality disorders, but also others when faced with acute stressors and a sense of losing control or feeling overwhelmed)

- Depression (especially if comorbid with any of the above)

Management of Violence or Imminent Violence

Perhaps the most important principle is first to ensure your own safety and (within reason) comfort. You cannot help your patient unless you are able to use your skills and mental resources freely and effectively. The bottom line, then, is to set limits on threatening situations, get out of the situation if setting limits is not possible or effective, and get additional help (staff, security, police) sooner rather than later if necessary.

In terms of the verbal interventions that may help defuse a potentially violent patient, you must walk a line between helping the patient feel empowered and understood (which may make him or her calmer and less prone to be violent) and setting clear limits on unacceptable behavior. To set limits, comments such as, "I'm not going to be able to help you unless you stop threatening me" or "You need to sit down and stop waving your fists in the air" may be entirely appropriate.

When patients actually are violent or otherwise losing control of their physical impulses, a "psychiatric code" is instituted. This involves:

- *Marshalling sufficient forces* (usually psychiatric staff plus security guards) to meet the situation.
- *Deciding on a specific plan of action* that is understood by the entire code team, such as,

"We're going to put the patient into four-point leather restraints on this stretcher bed and then administer an IM injection of lorazepam (Ativan) 2 mg." At this time it is important that explicit roles be assigned to each team member: "You will restrain the patient's left leg," or "I will give the injection."

- *Implementing the plan,* during which time the main verbal contact with the patient will consist of explaining *what* is to be done to him or her. Explanation of the *whys,* or answers to other patient questions, must await the completion of the code so that the patient and staff are safe from harm.

PSYCHOLOGICAL TRAUMA

In this context, trauma refers to the psychiatric consequences of exposure to life-threatening or otherwise unusually horrific situations. After experiencing events such as rapes, beatings, or physical disasters, persons vary widely in their responses: Some may become depressed, some may develop post-traumatic stress disorder (PTSD) or acute stress disorder, and others may develop other syndromes including mania, psychosis, anxiety, or somatoform disorders. Still others may not develop any diagnosable syndrome at all. Although the approach to the patient with recent trauma must vary depending on the details of the event and its context, common principles have emerged from research and clinical experience with several populations, including soldiers in combat; victims of earthquakes, floods, or other natural disasters; and rape victims. Essentially, the immediate use of brief psychotherapeutic techniques—building an alliance, using empathy and support, validating and encouraging the expression of thoughts and affects—will reduce acute symptoms, and probably reduce long-term complications as well. Patients must also be informed about the availability of ongoing psychiatric services and other relevant supports.

CATATONIA

Catatonia is a syndrome characterized by:

- Severe psychomotor abnormality, which may include:
  - Purposeless, self-directed, increased motor activity
  - Severe slowing or immobility; the latter may include catalepsy (a.k.a. waxy flexibility," in which limb position may be "molded" by the examiner, and the patient maintains this position)
  - Peculiar voluntary movements, including bizarre posturing, stereotypies, or other prominent mannerisms
- Mutism
- Negativism (resistance to all instructions or attempts at being moved)
- Echolalia (repeating others' phrases) or echopraxia (mimicking others' postures or movements)

Assessment

The differential diagnosis of catatonia includes:

- A variety of neurological conditions (e.g., encephalitis, vascular events, Parkinson's disease)

- Systemic conditions, most typically metabolic (e.g., hepatic failure, electrolyte disturbances)
- Medication side effects (e.g., neuroleptics)
- Idiopathic mood disorders (bipolar disorder, major depression)
- Schizophrenia
- Schizoaffective disorder

In patients newly presenting with catatonia, it may be difficult or impossible to tell whether delirium is also present. After all, how can you assess cognitive impairment, the hallmark of delirium, in a patient who is mute or resistant to commands and questions? However, given the above differential diagnosis, catatonia, like delirium, must be treated as a medical emergency until proven otherwise.

Management of Idiopathic Catatonia

Assuming that available current and past medical history, physical examination, and any relevant laboratory tests have failed to identify a specific cause for the catatonia, you must proceed to treat as if for an idiopathic psychiatric disorder. Most persons with de novo idiopathic catatonia ultimately turn out to have a mood disorder. A careful history of symptoms that were apparent prior to the full catatonic state, along with the psychiatric history of the patient and family, may be helpful.

Keys to management include:

- Supportive care, such as
  - Use of nasogastric or intravenous access to maintain adequate hydration and nutrition
  - Monitoring of vital signs
  - Care related to bladder and bowel function

- Attempts to prevent deconditioning by use of passive or active exercise

- Benzodiazepines: Oral or parenteral benzodiazepine administration (best described for lorazepam) may rapidly "lyse" the catatonic state. The underlying affective or psychotic condition remains, but supportive care and engagement with treatment are often much easier. For instance, the patient may now take fluids, food, and oral medications.
- Other drugs: Depending on the underlying episode and overall illness, neuroleptics, mood stabilizers, or antidepressants may be needed.
- Electroconvulsive therapy (ECT): Given its rapidity and great efficacy for mood episodes with psychotic features, ECT may be a first choice, although obtaining informed consent from a catatonic patient may be a bit of an obstacle to its use. (State laws vary, but in some places informed consent from next of kin may be used.)

MEDICAL EMERGENCIES OF DIRECT RELEVANCE TO PSYCHIATRY

Among the more common emergencies related to psychiatric disorders are physical trauma (including self-inflicted wounds), physical sequelae of substance intoxication or withdrawal, and intentional overdoses and self-poisonings. Management of these issues cannot be adequately discussed here, but is well covered in standard medicine, surgery, and emergency medicine references.

Some other specific medical emergencies are

related to psychotropic medications. We will briefly review three.

Acute Dystonic Reaction

The concept of dystonia as a side effect of traditional neuroleptics should sound familiar to you. (If not, take another look at Chap. 16.) It's useful to remember that other dopamine blockers that are not usually thought of as neuroleptics, such as prochlorperazine (Compazine) and metoclopramide (Reglan), may also cause dystonia.

Severe, acute dystonia occurs most often in younger people, especially men. Dramatic, uncomfortable, and potentially dangerous presentations may include:

- Torticollis (neck spasms)
- Opisthotonus (severe extension of the entire spine)
- Oculogyric crisis (fixed upward gaze)
- Laryngeal dystonia, which may lead to upper airway obstruction

Treatment of acute dystonia with intramuscular anticholinergics (or diphenhydramine if anticholinergics are not readily available) usually leads to rapid relief. Supportive measures, including securing an adequate airway in the case of laryngeal dystonia, should be used as needed until pharmacological relief has been obtained.

Neuroleptic Malignant Syndrome

NMS is a potentially fatal idiosyncratic reaction to traditional neuroleptics. NMS probably exists along a broad spectrum of severity. In the full-blown form, the symptoms include:

- Extrapyramidal side effects, especially rigidity
- Fever (may be quite high)
- Autonomic instability, which may include diaphoresis, wide fluctuations between low and high blood pressure, heart rate variability, or arrhythmias
- Delirium
- Seizures
- Skeletal muscle breakdown (due to severe rigidity), causing elevated serum creatine kinase levels
- Renal failure (due to myoglobinemia or hypoperfusion)
- Death (due to cardiovascular collapse, respiratory compromise, or renal failure)

The treatment of NMS may include:

- Discontinuation of all neuroleptics and other dopamine blockers
- Supportive care: hydration; cooling blankets; monitoring and management of cardiac, cardiovascular, and respiratory function; monitoring of renal function and dialysis when indicated; anticonvulsants
- Dantrolene, a muscle relaxant that may help with rigidity and consequent muscle breakdown
- Bromocriptine, a central dopamine agonist that may help the neurological components of the NMS syndrome

Anecdotal evidence suggests that patients with resolved NMS may successfully tolerate neuroleptic treatment, although usually an agent from a different chemical class is chosen. The decision to rechallenge with neuroleptics must weigh the severity of the NMS, the indications for neuroleptic treatment, alternatives to traditional antipsychotics (e.g., clozapine, risperidone), and the risks of not using neuroleptics at all.

Tyramine-Induced Hypertensive Crisis

We've already considered the symptoms of such a crisis, which may be the consequence of straying from dietary restrictions while taking a monoamine oxidase inhibitor (MAOI). The main treatment strategy is to control the malignant hypertension. Some physicians routinely give patients on MAOIs prescriptions for nifedipine, 10 mg capsules, and instruct them how to administer the antihypertensive sublingually in case of a crisis. In the emergency room setting, standard procedures for reducing blood pressure may be effective. In addition, use of alpha-adrenergic blockers may be particularly effective, since much of the hypertension is caused by peripheral vasoconstriction mediated by release of endogenous sympathomimetics. Phentolamine is the alpha blocker par excellence, but in a pinch, parenteral chlorpromazine (Thorazine) can be used.

19
CHAPTER

Other Essential (or at Least Interesting) Topics

This chapter is an even more varied grab-bag of topics that didn't fit neatly into other chapters.

LEGAL ISSUES IN PSYCHIATRY

There are many arenas in which psychiatry and the legal professions interact. Some of these issues will *not* be discussed here, including psychiatric malpractice, assessment of psychiatric damages or disability, and the insanity defense in criminal justice system proceedings. But rather than dwell on our omissions, let us proceed.

Competency, Capacity, and Informed Consent

In the United States, people are presumed to be able to exercise their rights as citizens unless proven otherwise. It takes legal proceedings, including a judge's decision, to declare a person "incompetent" and to take appropriate action from there, such as assigning legal guardianship, power of attorney, and so forth. As physicians, therefore, we cannot determine competency. What we *can* do is offer an expert opinion as to whether a person has a mental disorder that is affecting his or her ability to perform a particular act (making a decision regarding medical treatment, for example)—in other words, a mental disorder that is affecting his or her "capacity." In clinical treatment settings, the question of capacity arises most often hand in hand with the notion of informed consent for medical treatments.

Capacity is both time- and issue-specific.

Time. Capacity may change over time. For example, a delirious patient may be unable to make any reasoned decisions about care now but may fully regain his or her capacity when the delirium resolves. For this reason, all opinions about capacity are referent to the time of the examination, although you may certainly offer an opinion about the likelihood of change over time. For instance, in the case of an incapacitated, severely demented patient with Alzheimer's disease, you might state that further cognitive deterioration is to be expected and that, therefore, the patient is highly unlikely to regain capacity.

Issue. People's capacity may vary regarding different issues at the same point in time. For example, a delusional patient who (falsely, let's hope) believes that the doctor is trying to poison him may therefore lack capacity regarding the medications recommended. Yet he may be fully capable of managing his finances, or deciding on his place of residence at discharge, or voting for elected officials. (We'll avoid the obvious jokes here about his being more capable than most voters.) For this reason, all opinions about capacity should clearly indicate the relevant task or issue, such as "Ms. Xerxes does have the capacity to make an informed decision regarding the exploratory laparotomy that has been recommended to her."

Capacity depends on the ability to *understand* the issues at hand, as well as on the ability to make a *reasoned* decision. (Note that we did not say *reasonable* decision, which in practice is usually interpreted to mean, "Do what I would do.") Rather, is the patient able to think through the issues involved in order to arrive at, and defend, his or her decision? In the case of informed consent regarding a medical procedure, does the patient understand the problems faced, to a degree consistent with his or her education, intelligence, and cultural background? Does the patient understand the nature of the recommended treatment, its potential benefits, and its potential risks? Does the patient understand the nature, benefits, and risks of alternatives, including no treatment at all? Can the patient demonstrate how he or she thinks about these facts in giving, or refusing, consent for the procedure?

Of course, a patient's main source of information about his or her condition and treatment alternatives will usually be the health care providers. It is therefore crucial to take the time to describe and explain these data, using materials such as educational pamphlets when possible. To assess that the patient is truly giving informed consent, you must do more than ask, "Do you understand?" and accept the patient's nod as a "yes." Rather, you must ask patients to explain back to you how they understand what they have heard and how their understanding then leads to their decision about the procedure.

As physicians, and particularly as psychiatrists, we are often asked to decide whether a patient's capacity is impaired by a mental disorder.

Having a mental disorder is not enough, of course; most persons with psychiatric diagnoses still retain the capacity to make decisions about their care. Following are the most common ways in which capacity is impaired, arranged by broad diagnostic categories:

Psychosis. Delusions may affect a person's ability to either understand or reason through his or her medical circumstances (as in the previous example). A person who is too distracted by hallucinations or whose thought processes are too disorganized may also be unable to comprehend, retain, or reason appropriately.

Depression. An extreme example of the way in which depression may impair capacity is a patient who refuses lifesaving medical treatments because he or she wishes to die. In less extreme cases, depressive hopelessness, nihilism, or guilt may lead patients to refuse needed care. It is also not unheard of for hopeless patients to *accept* a procedure with the hope that it will bring death; this "consent" is certainly not "informed"!

Cognitive Deficits. Delirious, demented, or amnestic patients may not be able to comprehend or remember the facts relevant to a decision, or may lack the abstraction or frontal executive functions necessary to make an appropriately reasoned decision.

Some psychiatric diagnoses are *not* commonly accepted as grounds to declare that a patient lacks capacity. The most important of these are substance-use disorders and personality disorders. As clinicians, we recognize that these disorders certainly can distort or impair a person's ability to comprehend and process information or to make reasoned decisions, but broader legal and societal notions of "free will" usually take priority.

In practice, if a patient with severe borderline personality disorder refuses a medical recommendation, then even though we may recognize that this patient's pathology may have influenced the decision (through splitting or tendency toward impulsive actions), we would not opine that he or she lacked capacity to make an informed decision. Similarly, an alcohol-dependent patient who wishes to drink despite warnings of medical contraindications cannot be forcibly prevented from drinking. However, persons with these diagnoses may be prone to substance-induced or primary mood or psychotic disorders, which, if present, certainly might impair capacity.

Civil Commitment

Clinically, many patients in the acute phases of severe mental disorders will benefit from inpatient treatment. For some, inpatient treatment is the only alternative that can be expected to lead to clinical improvement or that will prevent them from harming themselves or others. Some of these patients will not want to be hospitalized, and some of the patients who refuse will do so out of impaired capacity. That is, the very mental illness that requires inpatient treatment may prevent the patient from making an informed decision about hospitalization. As well-intentioned clinicians, we might wish such incapacitated patients to be hospitalized against their will if necessary so that they can receive proper care.

From a legal perspective, this idea parallels the principle of *parens patriae*, the notion that government has obligations toward citizens unable to care for themselves. An additional principle is that of *police powers:* government may protect its citizens from harming one another, as in the physical assaultiveness of some acutely mentally ill patients. These two principles underlie the legal process of civil commitment, a specified mechanism that allows for the involuntary psychiatric hospitalization of certain acutely ill patients. The term "certain" is crucial, though, since principles of free will and autonomy are also important in our society; as a society, we do not wish to allow the indiscriminate use of involuntary hospitalization, even by well-intentioned health care professionals.

In reality, it boils down to the following: In most localities, involuntary hospitalization procedures are provided by state or local statutes. Often these statutes allow physicians (it may take more than one) to admit patients involuntarily for a brief period if the patients are judged to be dangerous to others or themselves. (The latter may include inability to care for their own needs.) Usually the court system is involved if the patient contests the admission or if a longer period of commitment is sought by the treating physicians. Many states also have statutes that formalize the status and rights of patients voluntarily admitted to psychiatric facilities.

Involuntary Medication

Clinically, it may make little sense to involuntarily hospitalize an acutely ill, dangerous, capacity-lacking patient and then allow the patient to refuse medications or other treatments needed to treat the acute state. From a legal perspective, however, involuntary treatment is a separate issue from commitment. Most states or other local jurisdictions have guidelines—statutes or local standards of practice—about how to handle situations in which a patient who is judged to lack capacity refuses medication. In some places, the clinician may take responsibility for care decisions, but most often, the matter must come to the courts before involuntary medications can be administered in all but the most emergent circumstances—and not even that exception applies in some states.

CHILD PSYCHIATRY

Child psychiatry is the medical specialty encompassing the diagnosis and treatment of mental disorders in infants, children, and adolescents. It has considerable overlap with the practice of general (and other subspecialty) pediatrics and adolescent medicine. There are also numerous areas of commonality of perspective and practice with general psychiatry, as exemplified by the training requirements: One must complete at least 2 years of general psychiatry residency training along with 2 years of a child psychiatry fellowship.

Compared with general psychiatry, there are also numerous differences, subtle and unsubtle, in the content and process of child psychiatry. The following is the briefest of overviews of such differences, a pre-orientation for those of you who (by choice or assignment) end up training in child psychiatry settings.

Developmental Issues

Attention to developmental issues is prominent in all of psychiatry, and indeed in all biopsychosocially sophisticated medical care, but it is an obvious inherent part of working with children, regardless of specialty. The biologic, psychological, and psychosocial changes over time in this population are rapid and profound. Children's capabilities and limitations at each level of conceptual organization are quite different, not only from adults but also from those of pre-adults of different ages. Developmental issues thus inform everything—differential diagnosis, psychodynamic formulation, interviewing techniques, treatment planning and implementation—and underlie the rest of the points to be made in this section.

Family

It should be apparent that most children are dependent on their families to a greater degree than most adults, and assessment of the family is crucial to almost all child psychiatric evaluations. Active involvement with the family is usually at least an important adjunct and can be the primary or sole treatment modality.

Social Systems

For similar reasons, nonfamily social systems are often crucial to the assessment, management, and (for severe cases) placement of child psychiatry patients. Such systems may include schools and other educational agencies, workshops and other vocational centers, residential facilities, child protective agencies, and so on.

Disorders That Are More Common in Childhood

A number of mental disorders, to use the *Diagnostic and Statistical Manual of Mental Disorders* (DSM-IV) phrase, are "usually first diagnosed in infancy, childhood, or adolescence." These are described below.

Mental Retardation. Defined as cognitive impairment with onset before age 18 years, mental retardation exists along a broad continuum of severity, so specifiers (e.g., "mild") are used, based on intelligence testing. Analogous to patients with adult-onset cognitive deficit disorders (see Chap. 4), patients with mental retardation may exhibit a wide variety of noncognitive psychiatric symptoms and syndromes.

Pervasive Developmental Disorders. These disorders are manifested by difficulties in several areas of development unrelated to intellectual deficits, including social interactions, communication skills, or stereotypies. Autism is perhaps the best known of these disorders among lay persons; other examples include Rett's and Asberger's disorders.

Attention-Deficit/Hyperactivity Disorder (ADHD). As implied by the name, ADHD is characterized by inattention along with impulsivity or motor hyperactivity. The lay press, and some antipsychiatry (or antipsychopharmacology) organizations, frequently point out the difficulties in distinguishing "normal" from abnormal symptoms in these realms. However, such heuristic notions— and the reality that diagnosis may be difficult in some cases— should not make us throw the baby out with the bath water (apologies for the choice of metaphor). ADHD can be an enormously impairing condition. At the same time, treatments (including psychotropics) can be quite helpful, often leading to substantial improvement in school or social performance.

Tic Disorder. Tics are defined as sudden, rapid, recurrent, nonrhythmic, stereotyped involuntary motor movements or vocalizations. Motor tics may be as simple as eye blinking or grimacing or may include more complex behaviors such as jumping, touching, or grooming activities. Vocal tics may range from sniffing or throat clearing to verbal utterances including coprolalia, the use of obscene or otherwise inappropriate words. Tics may be secondary to a variety of substances or medical/neurological conditions. A tic disorder is diagnosed if the tics are idiopathic. Diagnostic categories are defined by transience or chronicity and by the presence of motor or vocal tics. Tourette's disorder is defined by multiple motor tics *and* one or more vocal tics over a period of at least 1 year.

Other Disorders. Other disorders of children and adolescents include:

- Learning disorders
- Communication disorders (troubles with expression or reception of language)
- Conduct disorder (a pervasive pattern of disruptive, dishonest, or aggressive behaviors, often a precursor of antisocial personality disorder in adulthood)
- Oppositional defiant disorder (which may be a precursor of conduct disorder)
- Feeding or eating disorders of infancy or early childhood (e.g., pica)
- Elimination disorders (e.g., enuresis)
- Separation anxiety disorder (a relatively common entity that may develop in relation to life stress or significant losses and may be a precursor or harbinger of anxiety or mood disorders in adulthood)

Disorders Presenting Differently in Childhood

Most of the major disorders of adulthood, including psychotic, mood, anxiety, and somatoform disorders, may present during childhood. They may or may not differ in demographic or clinical characteristics in children. The following will serve as examples of potential differences.

Schizophrenia. Schizophrenia is uncommon in children, although the prevalence in adolescents approaches that in adults. (After all, peak incidence is in the late teens to early 20s.) However, children may manifest social withdrawal or eccentricities as a prodrome of schizophrenia. In such cases, schizophrenia may be suspected but cannot be firmly diagnosed until positive psychotic symptoms emerge; what in retrospect was a prodrome may at the time be difficult to distinguish from depression or other behavioral conditions. Full-fledged childhood schizophrenia must meet the same diagnostic criteria as for adults, except that the criterion of role dysfunction may be met by failure to achieve age-appropriate developmental advances rather than by an actual decline.

Depression. The incidence and prevalence of major depression in children and adolescents have been increasing, although at least some of the apparent increase may result from attitudinal changes leading to greater recognition of the illness, and willingness to treat it, by families and providers. The diagnostic criteria are the same as for adults, although in practice role dysfunction again may manifest as failure to achieve normal developmental goals. Also, in practice, children may be less likely than adults to overtly manifest the classic mood and ideational symptoms of depression, such as spontaneously exhibiting or complaining of sad mood, guilt, or hopelessness. The main overt indicators of depression in children may include irritability, boredom or disinterest, somatization, social withdrawal, or "acting out" behaviors.

Therapeutics

We have already noted the crucial role family therapy may play in the treatment of children and adolescents. We have also noted that interventions with and by social agencies, such as schools, may be a large part of the treatment strategies. Individual diagnostic or psychotherapeutic sessions with children are often organized around playing with toys, drawing, or other task-oriented activities used to allow patients to express feelings and thoughts that they might be unable to access solely by face-to-face verbal contact. (Indeed, similar principles underlie art therapy, music therapy, and other task-oriented work with adults.) Face-to-face talk therapy is used as appropriate and tolerated, particularly with older children and adolescents.

Pharmacotherapy is a useful adjunct for many patients, although it is probably the primary treatment far less often than in adult psychiatry. The basic principles of drug use in children are the same as for adults, including careful attention both to diagnosis and target symptoms. Unfortunately, patient, family, and societal attitudes toward psychotropic medications for children may be even more negative than for adults.

GERIATRIC PSYCHIATRY

In recognition of the growing body of knowledge and skills in this area, geriatric psychiatry has recently received official subspecialty status from the American Board of Neurology and Psychiatry. Successful practice of psychiatry with older patients requires a thorough grounding in general psychiatry, specific expertise regarding the mental disorders most common in later life, and some degree of knowledge and comfort with geriatric medicine, neurology, and gerontology. The following is a brief overview of some of the salient characteristics of the field.

Developmental Issues

The prominent developmental issues of later life underlie, or overlay, all clinical work with older patients. Often these issues relate to losses, including deaths, retirement, social isolation, and medical illnesses or functional disability in oneself and others. And, of course, the biggest issue of aging involves the need to prepare psychologically for one's own death; as part of this process, people will (at various levels of explicitness) perform "life review," a reexamination of their life's past events and meanings.

Family

Older persons are often closely engaged with, or dependent on, family members or other persons close to them, such as friends or neighbors. As with child psychiatry, contact with the family is essential to a full psychiatric assessment. In the case of the elderly, "family" often means adult children or grandchildren as well as spouse. Treatments often involve the family as an adjunctive or primary modality.

Social Systems

Again as in child psychiatry, assessment and treatment of older persons may involve a variety of agencies or social systems, including home health aides and visiting nurse services; a range of alternative housing options, from senior independent apartments to adult homes that provide greater supervision, to nursing homes that can provide skilled nursing care; psychiatric or dementia-oriented day programs; senior centers; meals-on-wheels programs; transportation services; and adult protective services.

Common Psychiatric Disorders in Older Persons

The most common new-onset psychiatric conditions in older persons include:

- Depressions (major depression and a variety of so-called "subsyndromal" states of clinically meaningful depressive symptoms that don't quite make the criteria for major depression).
- Dementia.
- Delirium.
- Psychoses (while most later-onset psychotic symptoms are due to the above three categories, some may be due to delusional disorders or include a fuller panoply of symptoms consistent with schizophrenia criteria).
- Secondary syndromes (see "Comorbidity" below).
- Other (including adjustment disorders and alcohol dependence). Note that new-onset primary anxiety disorders and somatoform disorders are quite *un*common in the elderly, although anxiety and somatoform *symptoms* may be common with the above diagnoses, and some people with chronic anxiety or somatoform disorders beginning in early or middle adulthood may still be symptomatic and need treatment in their later years.

Comorbidity

In younger adults, psychiatric comorbidity is common, as when mood and substance-use disorders exist simultaneously, each contributing to the other and making treatment trickier and prognosis poorer. In the elderly, *medical* comorbidity is the rule. This should not be too surprising; we're all familiar with the idea and the statistics of declining physical health with age. What's important here is that the systemic or neurological conditions of older age may often contribute to the onset and course of late-life psychopathology, either directly (e.g., by intrinsic brain disease such as Alzheimer's, or by systemic conditions that affect brain functioning) or by acting as stressors that affect a person's sense of self, family and other role functions, and so forth. The DSM-IV dichotomy between "primary" and "secondary" psychiatric syndromes is particularly problematic in the elderly. In practice, we must:

- Maintain a high level of suspicion for medical contributors when presented with new or worsened psychopathology in the elderly
- Maintain a high level of suspicion for psychiatric manifestations of medical illnesses, or for psychiatric contributions to somatic symptoms, frequent calls or office visits, noncompliance, and so forth
- Aggressively target and treat all potentially treatable psychiatric syndromes and medical conditions, recognizing their frequent interrelationships

Therapeutics

We have already noted the importance of family work in psychotherapy with older persons.

Group work can also be useful. Individual psychotherapy is viewed with more stigma by most older persons than by younger cohorts (this may change as the baby boomers age), but geriatric patients who accept referral often ally well with their therapists and can benefit greatly from flexible supportive/expressive approaches. In non-acute psychotherapies, therapists frequently assist patients with the life review process in the context of addressing symptoms and managing ongoing stressors and losses.

Pharmacotherapy in the elderly is complicated by several factors:

- Changes in drug absorption and metabolism related to age or to diseases associated with age may mean that lower doses are needed to reach a given blood level.
- Age-related changes in neurotransmitter activity make the older brain more sensitive to central nervous system (CNS) side effects of psychotropics (including tremor, ataxia, dysarthria, sedation, and delirium); this is especially true in persons with frank neurologic diseases.
- Variability increases with age, so the degree to which the above two points are true varies astonishingly in different older persons.
- Most published drug research has used relatively healthy or younger subjects. Treatment of the elderly, especially those with neurological or substantial systemic comorbidity, is often based on extrapolation from data obtained in other populations, or based on anecdotal evidence.

Suicide in the Elderly

We have already noted that older persons have the highest suicide rates. Older suicidal persons, as compared with younger persons, are more likely to intend to die and use methods of greater lethality. Of those elderly who do kill themselves, most have a diagnosable depressive disorder at the time of their death. Rarely have they seen a mental health professional, but most did see their primary care provider within a few weeks of their suicide. Therefore, public health efforts to reduce this significant cause of death in later life must begin with improved recognition and treatment of depression in primary care settings.

SLEEP DISORDERS

Despite common lay conceptions of sleep as nothing more than the absence of wakefulness, we now know that sleep is in fact a complex phenomenon involving a variety of neurological, systemic, and mental activities. You may recall that sleep is divided into rapid eye movement (REM) sleep, the state in which dreams take place (hence the choice for the name of the rock band), and non-REM sleep (has any band ever called themselves this?). Non-REM is divided into numeric stages based on sleep depth.

Altered sleep is a common symptom. It may be a sole symptom or part of a constellation of mental or physical findings. It may be due to a primary sleep disorder, caused by neurological or systemic disease or drugs ("secondary" sleep disorders), or caused by an idiopathic psychiatric disorder (e.g., the insomnia or hypersomnia of major depression).

Classification

Classification of sleep disorders has been confusing, at least in part because DSM-IV-style diagnoses have not always exactly matched the schemata proposed by others in the field. But the basic principles are fairly straightforward.

Insomnias. These are defined as difficulty initiating or maintaining sleep, or as nonrestorative (i.e., unrestful) sleep. They may be primary (idiopathic) or secondary (e.g., due to psychiatric disorders, drugs, physical conditions).

Hypersomnias. These are defined, obviously, as excessive sleepiness, whether manifested by lengthy "sleep episodes" (nighttime for most people) or by daytime sleepiness. Again, there are primary and a variety of secondary variants.

Other Dyssomnias. These include:

- Narcolepsy, which is manifested by
  - Irresistible attacks of refreshing daytime sleepiness
  - Cataplexy (brief episodes of sudden skeletal muscle atony)
  - Intrusion of REM sleep into the wakeful-sleep interface, as evidenced by hypnagogic or hypnapompic hallucinations, or by sleep paralysis while falling asleep or just awakening

- Breathing-related sleep disorders. Caused by ventilatory abnormalities that disrupt sleep, leading to complaints of insomnia, daytime sleepiness, or both, including:
  - Obstructive sleep apnea (upper airway obstruction occurs during sleep).
  - Central sleep apnea (cessation of ventilation without obstruction, presumed due to CNS factors).
  - Central alveolar hypoventilation (alveolar hypoventilation, such as that due to cor pulmonale, that is worsened during sleep).

- Circadian rhythm sleep disorder: sleep disruption caused by a mismatch between endogenous circadian rhythms and environmental cues or demands. Examples are "jet lag" or sleep disorders found in workers moving between night- and day-shift work.

Parasomnias. Defined as abnormal behavioral or physiologic events during sleep, specific sleep stages, or the transitions between waking and sleeping, these include:

- Nightmares (just what it sounds like—recurrent and distressing or impairing bad dreams)
- Sleep terrors (recurrent abrupt awakenings with the autonomic, and often affective, suggestions of "terror," but no dream is recalled, and later there is amnesia for the whole episode)
- Sleepwalking (pretty close to how it's often portrayed in the movies, except that the individual does not perform terribly complex tasks [e.g., murders] while sleepwalking)

UNEXPLAINED PHYSICAL SYMPTOMS (THE DREADED UPS)

It is quite common—indeed, in primary care settings perhaps the rule rather than the exception—for patients to present with unexplained physical symptoms. "Unexplained" may mean that there is no objective evidence of a known etiology or pathogenesis that could account for the symptoms, *or* that the symptoms are out of proportion to what would usually be expected from any known etiology or pathogenesis.

Differential Diagnosis

Patients, families, and physicians often suspect that psychiatric factors are the cause of unexplained physical symptoms. One should not assume that this is so, but it is certainly important to consider. Hence, the "psychiatric differential diagnosis" of UPS should include **"I don't know."** We must be willing to admit our ignorance. In the case of UPS, not only are we often ignorant, but there are good reasons to err on the side of presuming our uncertainty:

- Occult physical illness that later declares itself more definitively is common, as demonstrated by follow-up studies of patients diagnosed with "somatization" disorders, who show a high rate of subsequent diagnosis with neurological or other conditions
- Diagnosis of a psychiatric disorder depends not just on the *absence* of a physical disorder, but on the *presence* of specific clinical features consistent with the psychiatric diagnosis
- Taking a stance of ignorance may be useful in allying with the patient and managing his or her ongoing unexplainable symptoms, as described later in the discussion of treatment

Depression. We have noted before that somatic symptoms, or rumination about somatic issues, may accompany major depression. Successful treatment of the depression may eliminate, or greatly reduce, the patient's somatic concerns.

Anxiety Disorders. Again, we have noted already that anxiety may be accompanied by a wide range of somatic symptoms. For example, panic disorder is a common cause of referrals to cardiologists for chest discomfort. If a specific anxiety disorder is diagnosed, specific treatments may be indicated.

Somatic Delusions. A patient's somatic worry may reach delusional proportions; these delusions may occur in the course of several psychiatric disorders, including schizophrenia, schizoaffective disorder, delusional disorder (primary or secondary), mood disorders, dementia, and delirium. Treatments will be specific to the diagnosis. Please note, though, that unexplained pain is by itself not a delusion: Delusions must be falsifiable, and since pain is by definition a subjective experience, it cannot be proven untrue. However, a patient who insists that his or her pain is due to cancer, despite evidence to the contrary, *would* be considered delusional.

Psychological Factors Affecting Physical Condition. This is listed in DSM-IV and is certainly worth considering in our differential diagnosis here but is technically not a mental disorder. Rather, it is a way of recognizing that mental state can profoundly influence the course of disorders with known pathophysiologies. Common examples include the effects of psychological stress on diabetes mellitus, asthma, and idiopathic bowel hypermotility syndromes ("irritable bowel").

Malingering. In malingering, the patient consciously and willfully creates a symptom to achieve a specific primary gain. In other words, they lie, or "fake it." Common gains include money (in a lawsuit or a worker's compensation or disability claim); avoiding work; or getting out of jail, a prisoner-of-war camp, or some other undesired setting. Unless the patient admits to (or is caught) faking the symptoms, it can be difficult to distinguish malingering from a somatoform disorder.

Factitious Disorders. As in malingering, patients with these conditions consciously and willfully produce their symptoms. Often they create physical findings that require workup, such as "hematuria" by pricking their finger and putting a drop of blood into their urine sample. (Cases involving physical symptoms such as this are often referred to as "Munchausen's syndrome.") Unlike malingering, though, these patients are not aware of *why* they are doing this, and clearcut primary gains are usually absent. It appears that many of these patients are (unconsciously) using their falsified symptoms and signs to obtain nurturing from health care personnel or to express rage by "tricking" these personnel into unnecessary tests or procedures.

Somatoform Disorders. Most of the disorders in this category can be summarized as follows. The patient has one or more unexplained physical symptoms that cause significant distress, impairment, or seeking of medical attention. The symptoms are judged (by implication more often than by direct evidence) to be caused or exacerbated by psychological issues, often with attendant "secondary gain" such as increased attention from family. The symptoms are produced *un*consciously; that is, the patient is not aware of the connection between mental processes and the symptoms. For the patient, the symptom is entirely "real"; he or she is not "faking it."

The somatoform disorders are divided into somewhat arbitrary categories in DSM-IV, based partly on historical reasons. In fact, few clinicians in practice worry about these distinctions, but for the record they include *conversion disorder* (neurological symptoms), *pain disorder* (pain!), *undifferentiated somatoform disorder* (one or several symptoms not included in conversion or pain disorders), and *somatization disorder* (also known as Briquet's syndrome; these patients have chronic histories of multiple symptoms referent to several organ systems). *Hypochondriasis* is a disorder defined by illness worry and help-seeking alone (that is, without specific somatic symptoms); again, in practice few clinicians use this term with such precision.

The one somatoform disorder that may be different from the others is *body dysmorphic disorder*, defined as exaggerated worry without basis about a defect in one's appearance (e.g., the size or shape of one's nose, breasts, or genitals). These patients' worries may have an obsession-like quality, and the disorder may be more closely related to other Axis I disorders such as obsessive-compulsive disorder than to the other somatoform disorders.

Assessment

How to assess the patient with UPS? It is, of course, important to be clear that the patient's symptoms cannot be adequately explained by objectively demonstrable physical disease. This principle, however clear in theory, is not always easy to put into operation. Considerable clinical judgment is required to determine the extent of specialist consultation, laboratory tests, or other procedures required for a given patient with particular somatic symptoms.

It is also important to begin to explore the patient's psychiatric symptoms and psychosocial context as part of the initial and ongoing evaluation. Doing so facilitates rapid and accurate assessment and communicates to the patient that you take emotional factors as seriously as physical factors. Too often exploration of these dimensions is deferred until numerous tests have failed to reveal a clear physical etiology. Of note, as part of this history taking you will want to learn whether the patient has had any previous episodes of unexplained physical symptoms.

In considering psychiatric differential diagnosis, you will want to try to delineate disorders with the most specific treatments first: depression, anxiety disorders, and psychosis. If any of these is identified, education and discussion of treatment options should begin concomitant with any parallel physical workup.

If these psychiatric conditions are not present, and physical evaluation still leaves the patient's symptoms unexplained, you should have obtained enough sense of the psychosocial context to begin to speculate about somatoform or factitious disorders (and malingering). You also will have begun to build the alliance with the patient that will form the basis of management.

Treatment

Treatment of somatoform disorders, and of patients who somatize in the context of other disorders, is complex and difficult to summarize briefly. A few guidelines follow:

- *Do not* tell the patient that there is "nothing wrong" with him or her or that the somatic symptoms are "not real," "all in your head," or "due to" emotional problems. This advice may seem obvious, but too frequently physicians do communicate these notions to patients, either verbally or by not-so-subtle nonverbal cues. These attitudes destroy all hope of a useful alliance with the patient because they are so unvalidating of the patient's experience of distress.
- *Do* try to explore, in as nonjudgmental and open-ended fashion as you can, to what degree the patient believes the symptoms are

associated with or exacerbated by (not *caused* by) emotional factors. The patient's degree of openness versus hostility to such notions will help determine how quickly and aggressively (or not) you can expect to broach nonsomatic issues in your ongoing work together.

- Regarding the physical cause of the symptoms, *do* confess your ignorance. That is, tell the patient that you're honestly not sure what is causing the symptoms. At the same time, *do* offer reassurances that there is no evidence of a life-threatening illness or indications for further tests or other workup at this time. These statements must be combined with validating and empathic comments underscoring the patient's real distress.

- If the patient has no prior history of significant UPS, and the current symptoms are of recent onset, *do* offer encouragement as to the likelihood of spontaneous recovery in the near future. On the other hand, if the symptoms are chronic, *do* try to lower expectations; that is, convey that the likelihood that you will be able to fix the symptoms in the near future is low. But *do* offer encouragement that the patient may be able to function better, despite the symptoms, by not allowing the symptoms to dominate his or her life.

- If the patient is fairly open to the role of psychological or psychosocial factors, *do* begin to explore these issues in supportive psychotherapy, and consider referral to mental health specialists as indicated (and as accepted by the patient). If the patient is fairly hostile to discussion of these issues ("I'm not crazy, doctor, all I have is a physical problem"), you'll have to approach emotional issues in a much more oblique fashion (e.g., "Having this ongoing symptom must be stressful for you . . ."), and expect that it may take weeks or months to make much progress in openly addressing these issues together.

- *Do* see patients with chronic UPS at regularly scheduled appointments. This fosters the development of the treatment alliance, which may ultimately reduce their unnecessary utilization of health system resources and may reduce their symptoms as well. To put it another way, telling such patients to come back "if you need to" is an invitation for their symptoms or disability to worsen.

Index

A page number in *italics* indicates a figure. A "t" following a page number indicates a table.